THE
CONTRARIAN
DIET

THE CONTRARIAN DIET

LOSE WEIGHT EATING ICE CREAM, PIZZA, & CANDY

———

Joe King, G.E.D.

NOTICE

This book is intended as a work of humor only, and should not be misconstrued as a medical manual or nutritional advice. The information contained in this book can kill you. Read at your own risk.

This book may be unsuitable for persons who have no sense of humor or high literary standards. If either of these conditions persists, consult your physician. Following the advice of this book could lead to serious health problems including but not limited to explosive diarrhea, regurgitation, uncontrollable flatulence, severe bleeding of your retinas, excessive use of profanity, poor judgment, and not being able to fit in any of your clothing. Do not read this book while drinking alcohol or taking high doses of prescription medication, although doing so may enhance the enjoyment of the content of this book. Do not read this book while sleeping.

If you are a nutritional professional, attorney, or book critic that has nothing better to do than read silliness, note that many, or possibly all, references to the words "ice cream", "pizza", "candy", and other food throughout this book that may be deemed unhealthful could actually mean "celery", "broccoli", and "spinach", or other food. While this book discusses candy, the reader is reminded not to take candy from strangers.

The Contrarian Diet is not affiliated with the Salad, Soda, and Cigarette Diet. This book contains facts, many of which are completely made up. Any facts, opinions, or narratives contained herein are not necessarily true, and do not necessarily represent the views of any particular person. By reading this disclaimer you agree to hold the author, publisher, hostages, and anyone else involved in this book harmless.

Any spellling or grammatical errors in this book were made intentionally to annoy you. This book is not intended for Canadians. Reading this book backwards does not contain any subliminal messages, except for this... nrocpop yub. This book is sold by volume, not by quality of content. In the unlikely event that this book is turned into a movie, the reader agrees to inform everyone that the book was better than the movie, whether or not this is actually true. Keep book away from fire or flames, especially if you are reading this book in digital format as it may damage your Kindle or other reading device.

Dedicated to

the dieters that

faithfully support the

$60 billion dollar

a year industry

that can't solve

the problem

of weight loss.

CONTENTS
Note: Contents may have shifted during shipment.

PART I: UNDERSTANDING THE CONTRARIAN DIET

Chapter 1: LOSING WEIGHT, STOP EATING LIKE A COW 3
Chapter 2: A REALLY, REALLY BRIEF HISTORY OF DIETS 13
Chapter 3: GOOD SUGAR, GOOD CARBS.............................. 24
Chapter 4: SODIUM IS SODIUM GOOD 32
Chapter 5: GOOD FATS, THERE ARE NO BAD FATS 39
Chapter 6: ICE CREAM, AM I FAT YET?..................................... 45
Chapter 7: PIZZA, IS IT HEART DISEASE YET?................................. 52
Chapter 8: CANDY, IS IT DIABETES YET?....................................... 59
Chapter 9: LISTEN TO YOUR BODY.. 67
Chapter 10: BACK TO GASTROENTEROLOGY 81
Chapter 11: Why People Don't Fail on the Contrarian Diet 87
Chapter 12: How to Really Lose Weight... 91

PART II: MEAL PLANS & RECIPES

Meal Plan.. 95
The Contrarian Diet Recipes 103
CREDITS 176
GLOSSARY..177
About the Author 180

ACKNOWLEDGMENTS

Writing these acknowledgments is frustrating because it's impossible to mention all of the fads diets that have that have made this book necessary. Actually, it's not impossible. Let me list them for you:

The **Cabbage Soup Diet** for coming up with a weight-loss remedy that makes us fart.

Weight Watchers for convincing us to pay monthly fees for starving ourselves.

The **Slim Fast** diet for introducing us to the idea of milkshakes as diet food.

The **USDA** for pushing the low-fat diet in the 1980's that told us to eat more carbs and less red meat.

Atkins for pushing the low-carb diet of the 1990's told us to eat less carbs and more red meat.

Jenny Craig and **Nutrisystem** for helping us lose weight by making food expensive.

The **Raw Food Diet** for justifying eating cookie dough.

The **Zone Diet** for re-introducing us to fourth grade math by having us learn ratios and percentages all over again. Although, I still haven't figured out how we can eat a one pound box of chocolate and gain five pounds.

The **Mediterranean Diet** for creatively marketing us a diet that sounds more like a cruise than the torture of dieting.

The **vegetarian/vegan diet** which is simply a missed steak.

The **South Beach Diet** for inventing a diet that caused us to keep getting sand stuck in our teeth.

The latest craze, the **Paleo Diet**, for reminding us that the village idiot in prehistoric times that couldn't hunt, fish, or ride was called a vegetarian.

Food Poisoning for coming up with the quickest weight loss ever.

Exercising for making us think we lost weight, but then realizing our sweatpants came untied.

And all the other fad diets for providing us false hope through their schemes of temporary weight loss with a slim chance of losing weight long term.

If any one of these diets actually worked, there would be no need to continually come up with new fad diets... until now.

PART I:

UNDERSTANDING THE CONTRARIAN DIET

(THE NEW FAD DIET FOR PEOPLE WHO ACTUALLY LIKE FOOD)

Chapter 1

LOSING WEIGHT, STOP EATING LIKE A COW

"Be careful about reading health books. You may die of a misprint." - Mark Twain

"The first thing you lose on a diet is your sense of humor." - Unknown

The Contrarian Diet is not low-carb. It's not low-sugar.

It is not low-sodium either.

Nor is it low-fat.

The Contrarian Diet teaches you to eat a diet rich in sugar, carbs, sodium, and fat in the form of ice cream, pizza, and candy – and enables you to finally have a diet of the food you love. As a result, you're going to experience a dramatic weight change – somewhere between 5 to 20 pounds in the next several weeks.

Here's how you're going to do it.

First, you're going to stop eating like a cow. I know that sounds obvious when you're trying to lose weight, but that's exactly what most dieters do when they attempt to lose weight. Dieters start eating things like fresh veggies. That's the worst thing you could eat!

Every diet, except the Contrarian Diet, actually promotes the grazing on leafy greens. In restaurants, these things are politely referred to as salad. In nature, they are known as plants. In feedlots, they are called silage. Animals like cows eat them. Vegetables are the food that food eats. It's not what you should be eating.

Think about it. Eating like a cow is a bad idea. Cows are slow, lazy, and fat. How do you think they got that way? By eating ice cream, pizza, and candy? No, they got slow, lazy, and fat by eating salad (aka plants or silage).

If you don't want to look like a heifer, maybe you shouldn't eat what they eat. Put your salad fork down and stop eating like a cow.

People aren't supposed to eat like cows. Humans have evolved to the top of the food chain. The top of the food chain doesn't eat salad. The top of the food chain eats whatever it wants. We didn't fight our way to the top of the food chain to eat broccoli. We fought our way so that we could eat plates of nachos, large pizzas, and bowls of chocolate ice cream covered in whip cream. Don't let nutritionists, doctors, or other so-called health experts try to push you down the food chain by resorting to veggies. You're on top of the food chain and can eat anything and everything.

Welcome to the Contrarian Diet.

You've probably tried many other diets. Whether it's Weight Watchers, Zone, South Beach, Paleo, or anorexia, they pretty much all work the same way. They make you eat less to achieve short term weight loss and then you get frustrated, moody, hungry, and quit.

Don't blame yourself. Everyone who diets gains in the end. It's not your fault. These diets were designed to never work.

That's the brilliance of fad diets. They create temporary weight loss with no chance of long term success. After you drop a few pounds by starving yourself, you get frustrated and quit, and they know you'll be back again and again. The diet industry enjoys a heavy bottom line as they make tons of money selling you books, seminars, newsletters, cook books, diet scales, books, monthly meetings, and pre-packed diet foods. Did I mention they sell books?

These fad diets also disclaim their products and statements every time they claim it works because the Federal Trade Commission has sued them for deceptive trade practice. By the way, any statements in this book that claim the Contrarian Diet will help you lose weight or improve your health are hereby disclaimed as results are not typical.

The funny thing is that people claim that these diets actually work. You hear people say, "That diet has worked for me three times." Maybe they have a different definition of success than I do, but if you've been on it three times it sounds like that diet is a failure.

That's not the only illogical thing dieters do. The way people diet is the very definition of insanity: doing the same thing repeatedly but expecting different results. People keep going on diets that consist of fresh fruit and vegetables combined with aerobic exercise. After their current diet fails, they try another diet that consists of the same things: more fruit, veggies, and exercise.

Maybe you need to stop and ask yourself, if eating a diet full of vegetables and other allegedly healthful foods isn't working, shouldn't you try something new and completely different?

I know there are lots of medical doctors, nutritionists, and nagging mothers that say eating your vegetables is good for you. But what if they are all wrong? What if it's all a big fat lie?

If you've struggled with your weight your whole life, if you've tried dieting and exercising, if you've tried eating vegetables and still gained weight while your skinny friends ate bags of chips, if you're at your width's end, you're ready for a revolutionary change in the way you eat and the way you live. You need to try something different. Very different. Are you ready to try the complete opposite of what you've been doing? If you answered yes, then you're ready for the Contrarian Diet.

WHAT IS A CONTRARIAN?

The Webster dictionary defines a contrarian as "a person who takes the opposite or different position or attitude from other people." It also tells us that the word rhymes with barbarian, which is just a fun useless fact.

The word contrarian is often used in the investment world. Contrarian investing is done by people who invest in the opposite way as the rest of the people. These people are called contrarians, because they don't follow the herd. They do just the opposite. They try to make money doing so.

In dieting, the contrarian is also the person who goes against the herd. Contrarians don't eat silage like other dieters. They don't succumb to fad diets that push fresh veggies. Contrarians eat just the opposite of what other dieters eat. The contrarian eats a diet rich in sugar, carbs, sodium, and fat. They try to lose weight doing so.

I know what you're thinking. You think that food high in sugar, carbs, sodium, and fat isn't diet food; it's junk food. According to whom? The nutritionists that have recommended every diet you've previously tried and failed? Think about this... cows are big and fat. Cows don't eat cookies, peanut butter cups, pepperoni pizza, and double cheeseburgers (especially not cheeseburgers). They eat grass. Maybe those veggies aren't nearly as good for you as you were told. Maybe there's a reason you crave sugary, salty, fatty, yummy tasting food.

If you'd rather eat a slice of apple pie than an apple, keep on reading. The Contrarian Diet is for you.

Standard Diet Warning: Before starting any diet, including the Contrarian Diet, discuss the diet with your physician, your best friend, your co-workers, your co-worker's best friend, your mother, your neighbor, your co-worker's best friend's mother's neighbor, your Facebook friends, your Twitter followers, your favorite blog, and the next wrong phone number you dial to see if it's right for you. Second warning: Before discussing the Contrarian Diet with your physician, you may want to think it through. Asking a medical doctor permission to start a high-sugar, high-carb, high-sodium, and high- fat diet may not go over very well. Consider yourself warned.

THE CONTRARIAN DIET
The Contrarian Diet is like no other diet you've tried.

The Contrarian Diet turns the food pyramid on its head, and slops a second helping on top of MyPlate. It's based on the best research of leading scientists, nutritionists, and medical doctors. But, what makes the Contrarian Diet different is that it completely ignores and flies in the face of this research.

CONTRARIAN FOOD PYRAMID:

(Note that the Contrarian Food Pyramid has more of a smile shape than the traditional food pyramid.)

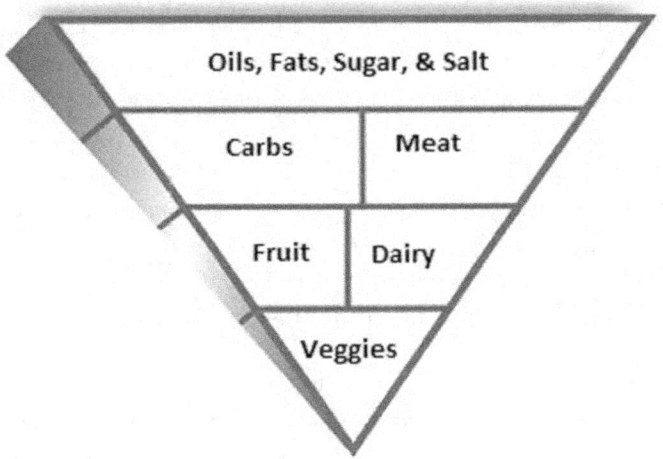

While other diets have unrealistic rules that are difficult and painful to follow, the Contrarian Diet is easy. There are no rules. You don't need to fear food. Rather, you embrace and enjoy food.

On other diets you may be hesitant to even look at the tempting food that the diet prohibits. On the Contrarian Diet, not only can you smell and look at delicious food, but you can actually eat the food in abundance. The Contrarian Diet isn't a diet of things you can't eat. It's a diet of what you can eat. Pizza and cheeseburgers aren't considered forbidden foods. Rather, they are the staples of the Contrarian Diet. You're not limited to little bite size portions either. You can eat all you care to eat.

On the Contrarian Diet, you will eat satisfying meals. The Contrarian Diet isn't a fad. It's about real change. By eating good, hearty food, you won't feel hungry, tired, or cheated on the Contrarian Diet.

For example, you may eat donuts for breakfast, macaroni and cheese for lunch, and a monster burrito and tortilla chips for dinner. And, yes, you can have your cake and eat it too.

You'll discover Power Foods on the Contrarian Diet, like ice cream, pizza, and candy. These are foods that taste good, are fulfilling, and provide your body the energy it needs. You'll discover some shocking and little-known nutritional benefits of these Power Foods later in this book.

Unlike other diets that eliminate entire food categories, like carbs or fats, the Contrarian Diet promotes them. The Contrarian Diet concentrates on sugar, carbs, sodium, and fat. The only food category that the Contrarian Diet discourages is vegetables. Even though vegetables are frowned upon, they aren't prohibited. For instance, it's fine to add lettuce and tomatoes to your burger if you desire. It's also acceptable to have green peppers on your pepperoni pizza, if that's what floats your boat. But you won't be forced to eat your vegetables or feel guilty if you avoid them. It's fine if you like to eat them, and totally fine if you'd rather have a bowl of ice cream.

The Contrarian Diet is about more than just weight change. It's also about health. Once you start the Contrarian Diet you'll notice major changes to your cholesterol, blood pressure, and sugar levels. Your health will change, and within months you'll need to buy a whole new wardrobe as your clothes will no longer fit.

The Contrarian Diet doesn't pressure you into exercising like other diets. Rather, the Contrarian Diet discourages exercise. You'll learn in a later chapter why exercise is bad for your health and why you should avoid it.

The Contrarian Diet is more than just a diet, it's a lifestyle. You'll be able to go out restaurants with friends and not worry about what to order. You'll be free to buy popcorn when you're at the movie theater. You'll be able to order a mocha with whip cream and whole milk in the morning, and even eat a donut if you want. You'll have the choice to have a pizza delivered if you're too tired to cook. You'll be able to hang out at the pub all night drinking if you've had a bad day. The Contrarian Diet will let you live a lifestyle that no other diet is able to offer.

Other than spending your hard earned money on this book, there is no nothing else you need to buy (except another copy for a friend). There is no diet food, no special boxes of prepared food to buy, no monthly meeting to attend, no need to weigh yourself, and no difficult list of do's and don'ts. There are no calories to count, no nutritional education required, no measuring food; you'll barely know you're on a diet. This is the easiest diet you'll ever be on. And you'll never want to quit.

If you've tried and failed at low-carb or low-fat diets, the Contrarian Diet is your answer. The Contrarian Diet isn't low anything, except low-failure rate. People have had great success with the Contrarian Diet as evidenced by the numerous fake testimonials throughout this book.

If you think this diet sounds too good to be true, just stop thinking, and tell yourself, "I deserve it!"

THIS SOUNDS ABSURD
Before you dismiss this diet as complete nonsense, ask yourself this: have any of the low-carb, low-fat, veggie pushing diets that you have tried in the past actually worked? Probably not if you're reading this diet book.

Maybe these diets are all taking the wrong approach. That's the beauty of the Contrarian Diet. It turns traditional diets on its head. If you can't lose weight avoiding sugar, carbs, sodium, and fat, why not try focusing on eating them instead and see if it works. You have nothing to lose, and a lot to gain.

While you may think that the Contrarian Diet is absurd, it's no more ridiculous than the other popular diets that are on the market today. One of the most popular fad diets currently is suggesting that people should eat like cavemen. How can anyone take that seriously? Any diet that tells you to only eat limited types of food and avoid others is absurd. The Contrarian Diet doesn't limit what types of food you eat. Plus, if you're going to go on a diet, it might as well be one that is fun and one that you'll be able to enjoy good food.

FAKE TESTIMONIAL #1
LAURA LYNN HARDY: **I STARTED THE CONTRARIAN DIET AND GOT A DATE TOO**

I had just returned home to Miami Beach from a long vacation in Vegas. I had put on a few extra pounds, like 40 or so. You know eating at all those salad buffets along the Vegas strip. I didn't want any food to go to waste.

When I got back from vacation, I weighed 165 pounds. Sure, I might have been a tiny bit overweight, but it was all vacation weight, which doesn't really count anyway. But I did know that I needed to address my recent weight gain, so I avoided things that made me look fat, like mirrors, scales, and photographs.

One day I heard a knock on the door. I asked, "Who's there?"

I heard a voice say, "It's the UPS man."

"UPS man who?" I replied.

"Look lady, this isn't a knock knock joke! Open the door. I have a package for you."

I opened the door and there stood a tall, fit UPS man. He looked so handsome in his UPS uniform. Our eyes met and his hand brushed my hand as he handed me a small box. I was in love.

I stood in my doorway admiring him as he walked back to his truck and drove away. Once he was gone, I went inside and looked at the box he had given me. It was addressed to me, but funny thing was… there was no return address.

I opened up the box and discovered a copy of the Contrarian Diet. Who would mail me a copy of a diet book anonymously?

I wasn't fat. How could I have been? I was a vegetarian. I ate tofu. When I first became a vegetarian I had to answer a lot of the hard questions that people face when they make that choice. As a vegetarian, should I eat animal crackers? If we aren't supposed to eat animals, why are they made out of meat? I didn't have the answers to those tough life questions.

The other question I still couldn't answer was who would send me a diet book? Then it hit me. Maybe the anonymous gift was from a secret admirer. Maybe it was the UPS man. Maybe the UPS man wanted me to get skinny so I could be his girlfriend. I got so excited! I read the entire Contrarian Diet book.

I followed The Contrarian Diet's advice and started eating sugar, carbs, sodium, and fat. I ate cheeseburgers and fries, and drank soda and milkshakes like I didn't care about life. My girlfriends stopped spending time with me once I started the Contrarian Diet. No, it wasn't because I smelled like a deep fryer, although I don't think that helped. It was because I couldn't stop talking about the new man in my life.

When my mother heard I was on a new diet and saw all the food I could eat, she got on The Contrarian Diet too. Unfortunately, she passed away shortly after starting the Contrarian Diet. She was 48. Although, I don't think it had anything to do with the diet. I'm still convinced it was natural causes. That's another reason I quit eating natural foods.

I still don't know who sent me the Contrarian Diet, but I don't really care. It helped me start dating the UPS driver. While technically we aren't dating, I order a copy of the Contrarian Diet ever week so I'm seeing the UPS man on a regular basis now.

Sure, I would love to lose a bunch of weight, but not as much as I'd like to date the UPS man. The Contrarian Diet has allowed me to eat whatever I want and see the UPS man every week. I can't understand how I was living without the Contrarian Diet and my weekly dates with the UPS man. I couldn't have asked for more than this.

Note: Individual experiences while following the Contrarian Diet are unique and may vary for each individual dieter. The testimonials listed in this book are fictitious and, like any fad diet, are not typical. Starting the Contrarian Diet most likely will not get you a date with the UPS man, or any man for that matter. Testimonials, reference and/or results do not guarantee or predict future results, and you should not specifically expect to experience these results. Basically, these testimonials serve the sole purpose of deceiving you to feel good about yourself and give you a false sense of potential success on the diet.

Chapter 2

A REALLY, REALLY BRIEF HISTORY OF DIETS

"I tried every diet in the book. I tried some that weren't in the book. I tried eating the book. It tasted better than most of the diets." - Dolly Parton

"In the 1960s, you could eat anything you wanted, and of course, people were smoking cigarettes and all kinds of things, and there was no talk about fat and anything like that, and butter and cream were rife. Those were lovely days for gastronomy, I must say." – Julia Child

From the beginning of humanity, people have worried about food. But not like people do today. Rather, they worried about how they would get enough food. Any food.

Back when people wore fur clothing, carried clubs, and lived in caves, they didn't think too much about what food they ate for dinner. If they could find it, or catch and kill it, they ate it. If it tasted good, or if they were hungry, they ate more of it.

These cavemen didn't worry about the amount of cholesterol they were eating from large slabs of raw red meat they ate. They never looked for a nutrition label on the outside of the Woolly Mammoth that they were going to eat, probably since there wasn't one and even if there was they couldn't read it. They didn't turn their backsides when they came to a lake to see if their butt was too big. And they didn't run around outside the cave wasting calories for the sole purpose of trying to slim down.

In fact, these cavemen racked their small brains trying to invent the wheel so they wouldn't have to walk. They desired high fat, high calorie meals. They'd kill with their bare hands to get it. Maybe they'd use a spear, but you get the point.

These people are our ancestors. That's right; we all come from a line of blood-thirsty, over-eating, lazy, illiterate, barbaric group of people. It's in our DNA.

As people progressed, the way people ate pretty much stayed the same. Yes, people did change from hunter/gatherers to farming since they were lazy. However, people ate whatever they could find, grow, or shoot. They didn't obsess over being skinny. They didn't worry about what food they ate.

People ate food pretty much in this same fashion for tens of thousands of years. People ate sugary food, salty food, and fatty food. 100 years ago butter and sugar were considered good for you. People ate bacon and eggs for breakfast. They used white bread to make sandwiches covered in butter or cheese and meat. They drank beer and whisky.

Life was good.

In the 1960's and 1970's, everything changed.

FEAR AND HATE: SUGAR, SALT, AND FAT

Through a combination of bad scientific studies, hypothesis sold as truth, bad public policy, and good old-fashioned public fear mongering, the public began a fear and hatred of sugar, salt, and fat. Before the 1960's, sugar, salt, and fat were considered food. Now, they were being portrayed as poison.

The public bought into this new research and avoided sugar, salt, and fat. A nation of sugar-a-phobes, salt-a-phobes, and fat-a-phobes was created as hate and fear swept the land. With this hate for sugar, salt, and fat, industries were brought to their knees and entire food lines were slaughtered to the point of extinction.

Remember Mister Salty Pretzels? Eating salt was considered normal when this product was introduced on the market. People used to politely ask, "please pass the salt" at dinner tables across America. Nowadays, asking someone to please pass the salt is like asking someone to please pass the meth. It wouldn't be considered good table manners. After 30 years, Mister Salty was pulled from the market by Nabisco in the 1990s because the public had become so salt-a-phobic.

Sugar Crisp suffered a similar fate. The sugary breakfast cereal was launched in 1949, back when eating sugar was socially acceptable. Women in the 1940's and 1950's weren't labeled bad mothers for feeding their children sugary cereal for breakfast. That's changed now. Sugar Crisp had to be re-labeled as Golden Crisp. Thanks to the sugar-a-phobes, many sweet cereals have either gone off the market or have had to drop the word sugar from their title, or even worse drop the level of sugar in their ingredients.

The sellers of fatty food have also been forced to hide in shame. Kentucky Fried Chicken and Dairy Queen were forced by the pressures of society into name changes. Like the other phobias, fat-a-phobia also swept the country. Kentucky Fried Chicken tried to distance itself from fatty fried foods by changing their name to Kitchen Fried Chicken, which never caught on, and then to KFC. Dairy Queen also ashamed of their fatty food, tried to distance itself from ice cream by re-naming the chain DQ.

While many will claim these dietary shifts away from sugar, salt, and fat are "good for us", where is their proof? They certainly don't make food taste any better. In the 1980's, when McDonalds changed from frying French fries in animal fat to vegetable oil, the new French fries didn't taste as good. In the early 2000's, when Starbucks got rid of pastries with trans-fat, their morning treats lost their tastiness. Clearly, the anti-sugar, anti-salt, anti-fat movement didn't improve the taste of food.

What about health? Did all of the sugar, salt, and fat hating help people become healthier? Nope, the movement didn't improve that either. Americans are fatter than ever. Look at old photographs before the 1960's. Everyone is skinny. Look around at the people today. Almost everyone is overweight. I know that doesn't make sense, right? If over 50% of the population is obese, then we're no longer overweight. We're average.

So if the fear and hate movement of sugar, salt, and fat doesn't make food taste better, and it doesn't make Americans healthier, what is the benefit?

We're lead to believe that we will live a much longer life.

The idea is that you will suffer now eating vegetables and things that taste disgusting. You'll abstain from eating yummy sugary, salty, and fatty foods. You'll exercise like crazy. By going through this suffering your whole life, you'll live longer so you can continue to eat crappy tasting food and sweat like a pig as you exercise.

If you don't buy into this plan, the so-called experts claim that you'll have a premature death. Is this actually true? Do we have any proof that eating sugar, salt, and fat will put us in the grave earlier?

Most of us think that answer is obvious. Yes! People before the 1960's died in their 30's and 40's back then, that's why we diet, right? Wrong.

This may be a shocker, but people lived about the same back then as they do now. Our modern diet doesn't make us live longer. The modern day low-sugar, low-sodium, low-fat diet crazes don't actually improve our lifespans. The promise of a longer life through healthful eating is a big fat lie.

While many of us believe people died early in life in the past because of their poor medical practices and diet, it's not as true as you'd think. There is no scientific evidence that our lifespans have increased by any significant amount over the last couple thousand years. I know that sounds a lot like there is no scientific evidence that smoking causes lung cancer. But, let's look at the facts.

Part of the misconception that humans are now living longer is due to the confusion over the terms lifespan and life expectancy. Life expectancy isn't the age that people are expected to die. It's just an average. This has been increasing. The Centers for Disease Control and Prevention states that life expectancy is now around 78 years. According to the National Center for Health Statistics, life expectancy for men has been improving over time. In 1907 life expectancy was around 45 years, in 1957 it increased to 66 years, and by 2007 it increased to over 75 years.

As you can see, life expectancy has been increasing. However, it isn't the change in diet that has caused it to increase. It was the improvement in the infant mortality rate. In 1907, the infant mortality rate was nearly 10 percent. In 1957, it improved to 2.6 percent. In 2007, infant mortality was under 1 percent.

Life expectancy is just the average age people lived. It doesn't tell us how long a person is expected to live. If one person dies at birth and the other lives to be 90, the average life expectancy of this group is 45 years. But that doesn't really tell you how long someone is expected to live. It's just an average. People weren't dropping dead in their mid-40's in 1907. The life expectancy number is skewed by the high infant mortality rate.

Lifespan, unlike life expectancy, has remained about the same for thousands of years.

People a hundred or two hundred years ago didn't eat prepared diet foods, count points, or eat and drink low-fat products. They did eat things like pies and cakes, fatty cuts of salted meat, and pizza and pasta. They ate food high in sugar, carbs, salt, and fat. They considered it real food, not junk food. They didn't feel guilty about it. And from what science tells us, they didn't die a premature death because of it.

To sum up the conventional wisdom as it pertains to diet and health, if you eating veggies and exercise regularly, the only benefit you'll receive is that you'll die healthier.

A RUN DOWN ON THE POPULAR DIETS
Every fad diet throughout history has a common theme. Diets make you fat. Also, they all focus on the fear and hate of sugar, salt, and/or fat. Let's take a quick trip through the history and misery of these diets.

1820- THE VINEGAR DIET
British poet, Lord Byron, popularized the vinegar diet. He would drink large amounts of vinegar and water to cleanse his body. He also ate potatoes soaked in vinegar. He did lose weight, although it was due to malnutrition, vomiting, and diarrhea.

EARLY 1900'S - THE FLETCHERISM DIET
Horace Fletcher, an overweight San Francisco art dealer, came up with a technique called "Fletcherism" after he was declined health insurance. He developed a technique of chewing each mouthful of food for at least 32 times, once for each tooth, and then splitting it out. It was kind of like bulimia without the vomiting. He thought that he would absorb the nutrition of the food without actually eating it. Fletcher did lose 40 pounds,

and his diet swept the nation. Fletcher's technique of counting the number of times you chew was soon replaced by a new diet technique called counting calories.

1920's – TAPEWORM DIET
The idea behind this diet is that you would swallow a pill with a tapeworm cyst. The tapeworm would live in your intestine and help consume the food you ate. Rumor has it that opera singer Maria Callas dropped 65 pounds in the 1950's on the Tapeworm Diet.

1928 – THE CIGARETTE DIET
Before the Surgeon General warning, tobacco companies made many claims about how smoking could improve your health. In 1928, Lucky Strike cigarettes launched an advertising campaign targeting women with advertisements that read "Reach for a Lucky instead of a sweet." Another advertisement read "Light a Lucky and you'll never miss sweets that make you fat." The campaign was very successful, however Lucky had to end the campaign after the candy industry threatened litigation. Later the candy cigarette was invented and everyone was happy.

1930's - THE GRAPEFRUIT DIET
Also known as the Hollywood Diet. The idea behind the grapefruit diet is that grapefruit allegedly burns fat. So does gasoline when it's lit on fire, however I don't advise drinking gasoline. On the grapefruit diet you eat a boat load of grapefruit and hope it burns your fat away.

1950's - THE CABBAGE SOUP DIET
The goal of the cabbage soup diet is to lose 10 pounds in a week eating cabbage soup. You can eat as much cabbage soup as you want. That's kind of like saying you can eat as much grass clipping as you want. Of course you're going to lose weight. You won't want to eat any cabbage soup. The side effects of the cabbage soup diet, other than losing water weight, are severe bloating and flatulence. If you're trying to slim down and drop a quick 10 pounds a week before a wedding, it may not be a good diet as you'll stink up the room like a dairy farm.

1954 - HCG DIET

This diet involves being injected with Human Chorionic Gonadotropin (HCG) from pregnant women's urine. Supposedly the HCG suppresses appetite (consuming urine normally does). Dieters on the HCG diet are limited to 500 calories a day. In 2011, Snooki brought this diet back into popularity.

1963 - WEIGHT WATCHERS

Jean Nidetch liked to eat cookies and soon weighed over 200 pounds. After being asked when she was due, she decided to invite some overweight friends to her apartment to talk about dieting. As the women lost weight together, soon they were able to squeeze more women inside her apartment. In 1963 she officially launched Weight Watchers International.

1964 - THE DRINKING MAN'S DIET

The original diet was invented by William the Conqueror in 1087. The king was so fat that he couldn't ride a horse anymore. The king decided to cut back on food and just drink alcohol. The diet worked and he lost weight. In 1964, a similar diet was introduced by Robert Cameron who published a pamphlet called "The Drinking Man's Diet" that sold 2.4 million copies. It's a low carb diet, similar to Adkins or South Beach, except you can drink whisky like a fish.

THE 1970'S - PROLINN DIET

Robert Linn, MD, invented a diet called the Prolinn Diet or The Last Chance Diet. He advocated not eating anything except Prolinn, which was ground animal hooves, horns, tendons and bones. Millions of people tried it. 58 people on the diet suffered heart attacks. Years later Robert Linn confessed that it was just an April Fool's Joke. Actually he didn't, but it seems like some kind of sick joke.

1970 - THE SLEEPING BEAUTY DIET

This diet was pure genius. Just sedate an overweight person for several days so they can't eat and let them starve while they're sleeping. Elvis is rumored to have tried the sedation diet. He hasn't been seen since.

1972 – ATKINS DIET

Dr. Atkins published Diet Revolution in 1972. In 2002, he published New Diet Revolution. The diet became very popular as people could finally justify eating bacon. Plus, the Adkins diet was the first diet that men thought was cool. Dr. Atkins medical report showed he weighed 258 pounds at death and had a history of heart attack and congestive heart failure.

1977 – SLIM FAST

Slim Fast comes up with the plan of a shake for breakfast, a shake for lunch, and then a sensible dinner. The idea of drinking shakes as meals is great, but I prefer real milkshakes.

EARLY 1980S – AYDS

A candy that suppresses appetite called Ayds was marketed. Ayds was taken off the market in the early 1980's during the AIDS crisis. Apparently no one wanted Ayds.

1995 - THE ZONE DIET

Biochemist, Barry Sears, comes up with the Zone Diet, a 40-30-30 ratio of carbs, fat and protein. Despite the need to do math, you do get to eat five times a day.

2003 – THE SOUTH BEACH DIET

Arthur Agatston, MD, comes up with the South Beach Diet. While the diet is just a mix of the Atkins and Mediterranean diets, the real women of South Beach maintain a diet that consists of moving their food around their plate with their fork, drinking cheap wine, and smoking cigarettes.

2010S – THE PALEO DIET

The Paleo diet reverses 10,000 years of human progress, and somehow makes eating like Fred Flintstone trendy.

2013 - THE COTTON BALL DIET

Models swallow cotton balls as a meal substitute. Some dip them in juice or gelatin for a little flavor. They're high in fiber and are supposed to be filling. I guess that gives a whole new meaning to the saying, "I'm stuffed" after you finish a meal.

FAKE TESTIMONIAL #2
KENNY DEWITT: **I NEVER FEEL HUNGRY ON THE CONTRARIAN DIET**

You could say I'm a serial dieter. I've tried all the fad diets. Most of them left me hungry. That's why I did Jenny Craig and Weight Watchers at the same time because I knew I wouldn't get enough food on just one diet.

I had gained some weight and decided it was time for a new diet. Everyone I knew was trying the Paleo Diet, so I decided to try it as well. I thought it would be fun to live like a caveman. I knew I couldn't eat processed food anymore, so I committed myself to hunting and gathering.

I wanted to do the Paleolithic diet the right way. The way our ancient ancestors actually ate. My plan was to hunt and gather my own food. It was first thing in the morning, so I thought I'd start this diet right away. I also wanted to look the part. I thought I'd make some fur clothing out of the first animal or two that I killed. In the meantime, I just stripped down to my undies. That's as close to a caveman as I could get.

I started by heading to the woods behind by house. I found a large, thick piece of wood about two and a half feet long. It would make a perfect club. I also found a heavy stick that was slightly bowed that I could use as a bow. The problem with the bow is that I didn't have anything to use as a bowstring. Also, it's actually very difficult to find straight sticks in the woods, and even if I could find any I didn't have a way to sharpen the arrows.

With a club and a useless bow, I began my hunt. It was around noon so I was hungry for lunch. I had my hefty club in my right hand and my bow in my left hand. I was ready to kill anything that moved. After looking for about 20 minutes, I couldn't find any animals. There were plenty of birds, however. I wasn't too worried about how the bird would taste. It would probably just taste like chicken, right?

I spotted a crow that was standing on the ground, so I slowly crept up on it. As I got closer, it would just fly further away. Not being able to shoot an arrow, I threw my bow at the crow. My bow didn't even make it half way to the bird. This hunting thing was going to be much more difficult than I had imagined. I threw my bow at a couple more birds and then called it quits.

I put the bow down and thought I'd give the club a try. I hadn't eaten all day so I was getting hungry. I thought I'd keep looking around the woods and see if I could find an animal. After looking for over an hour, I spotted a rabbit. That would make the perfect Paleo meal! Since by bow was ineffective, I thought I would sneak up on the rabbit and bash it repeatedly with my club.

I slowly crept up on the rabbit. I'm pretty sure it could see me because it looked really nervous. I guess I would be too if some hungry guy only wearing underwear and holding a big club was sneaking up on me. As I crept closer, the rabbit took off hopping. I guess I got a hair too close. Boy could that rabbit hop fast! I took off after it running as fast as I could. The rabbit was just too fast and got away. For the first time in my life, I didn't like fast food. The alternative to eating fast food would be to find a snail, but I really don't care for French food.

I was starting to see how this Paleo Diet worked. You lost weight because you couldn't kill any food. It was getting to be late afternoon and I still hadn't eaten. I thought I'd give foraging a try. I went back into the woods and starting looking around at the ground to see what I could find.

I was hoping I'd get lucky and find a berry bush, a mushroom, or perhaps a cheeseburger. Wait, I can't eat processed food. Strike the cheeseburger. I needed to find some berries, mushrooms, or nuts.

I looked around for what seemed to be hours. I didn't see anything other than trees, poison ivy, pinecones, moss, and a couple empty beer cans. I seriously thought about eating some bark and moss. Just about then, I saw a neighborhood cat. No, I wasn't going to kill the cat. However, I figured the cat was probably out in the woods hunting as well. I'd just follow it around and let it kill the food and then I'd scare it away with my club. So, I followed the cat around. It would occasionally freeze, crouch down and watch a bird. Then it would continue stalking in the woods. It seemed like the cat had just as hard of a time hunting as I did. Maybe the cat was on the

Paleo diet too. I was getting really hungry and tired. I decided to take a nap under a tree.

When I woke up, it was starting to get dark outside. Now I was hungry and cold. I thought I better either go home or start a fire. I didn't want to quit on my first day of the diet, and I needed a fire just in case I caught an animal. I found several rocks, some dry grass, and a couple sticks. I arranged the rocks on the ground in a little circle to make a fire area. Then I put the dried grass in the middle and started rubbing the two sticks together over my newly constructed fire pit. I rubbed and rubbed the sticks together, but no fire. Not even a spark or any smoke.

I was alone in the woods, almost naked, cold, and extremely hungry. I had to admit that I didn't have the primitive skills necessary to make effective weapons or even make fire. If I had to rely on eating like a caveman, I would be dead soon. I decided to quit the silly Paleo diet.

I walked home in defeat. I called for pizza delivery and drank a couple beers. I thought, this is the perfect diet. I want to find a diet where I can sit in the comfort of my home, eat pizza, and drink beer. I found out later that there was a diet like that. It's the Contrarian Diet, and I've been on the Contrarian Diet ever since. I'll never go hungry on the Contrarian Diet.

Chapter 3

GOOD SUGAR, GOOD CARBS

"I don't want to live in a world where I have to eat sugar-free sugar cookies." – Animal Crossing: Wild World (Nintendo Video Game) Written by Takayuki Ikkaku

"Only when you have eaten a lemon do you appreciate what sugar is." – Ukrainian Proverb

I'm not a diet doctor. I'm a gastroenterologist.

I spend most of my time listening to old people complain about constipation. But that has nothing to do with my job. I'm not a real doctor, I just play one in books. But if I were a real doctor, I'd help people lose weight by eating sugar and carbs.

Sugar is part of the trifecta of most hated and feared foods: Sugar, Sodium, and Fat.

In the world of dieting, sugar and carbs are public enemy number one.

Let's start by looking at sugar. Of all the food, sugar is both feared and hated the most. People hate sugar. Doctors hate sugar. Dieticians, dentists, school boards, and government policy makers all hate sugar. Mothers hate sugar.

However, we all love the taste of sugar. Every year, Americans eat an average of 150 pounds of sugar. Yet, we fear that sugar is bad for us. Many would even say sugar is the worst thing we can eat. Where did this hatred of sugar come from? Why are we so afraid to eat sugar?

It all started in 1972. A book titled "Sweet and Dangerous" written by Professor John Yudkin launched a public scare of sugar after he claimed that sugar was linked to heart disease. In 1988, he followed up with another book titled "Pure, White, and Deadly." No, that book wasn't about Ronald Reagan; it was another book about the evils of sugar.

Since the 1970's, sugar has become feared and hated as the so-called experts have claimed that sugar causes obesity, diabetes, heart disease, and global warming (maybe not the last one). Other than the great taste, people think that there is absolutely nothing good about sugar. Sugar is addictive. It's called poison and "kiddie cocaine." Sugar just makes you fat, hyper, and prone to cavities, diabetes, and heart disease. Basically, people think sugar is evil. And no one wants to be a fat, toothless, hyperactive diabetic about to have a heart attack.

But sugar wasn't always viewed as evil. A hundred years ago sugar was a staple in the American diet. People ate and enjoyed sugar. Why shouldn't they? People have been enjoying sugar for thousands of years.

Sugar is a natural food that comes from both sugar cane and sugar beets. Sugar is native to India and was originally consumed by chewing on the sugar cane.

In ancient times, people outside of India used honey as a natural sweetener. When Darius went to India, the Persians discovered a reed that "gives honey with the aid of bees." Sugar was traded throughout the Middle East and into Egypt and Rome. Sugar was a rare and valuable spice. It was used both for medicinal purposes and for cooking.

When people arrived in the New World, they brought their love of sugar with them. Sugar plantations were setup in the South and the Caribbean islands to keep up with the demand for sugar.

People have been eating and enjoying sugar for centuries and centuries. Did people have it wrong about sugar all this time?

No. Sugar is a necessary and an important part of a healthy diet. The paranoia about sugar that has been created by scientists, nutritionists, and government policy makers over the last several decades is unhealthy.

Sugar Myths De-Bunked

There are a lot of myths and misinformation about sugar. The first myth is that sugar is fattening. This isn't true. Sugar only has 15 calories per teaspoon. Sugar is no more fattening than any other food that has 15 calories. Sugar is a carbohydrate, which the body quickly converts into energy.

You probably think sugar is unnatural. Sugar is found naturally in fruits and vegetables. Sugar cane and sugar beets have the highest concentration of sugar. Sugar is made by extracting it from the sugar cane or sugar beet plant. The sugar, or sucrose, from either of these plants is identical. The sucrose from sugar cane is also identical to the sucrose in fruits and vegetables.

You also probably think sugar is unhealthy. Sugar is part of a healthy diet. According to the Sugar Association, which has absolutely no bias when it comes to the nutritional value of sugar, "carbohydrates, including sugar, are the preferred sources of the body's fuel for brain power, muscle energy and every natural process that goes in every functioning cell."

You may also think that going on a sugar binge will cause you to go into a diabetic coma. That's not true. Eating sugar doesn't cause diabetes. Ask any trick-or-treater.

Health Benefits of Sugar

Sugar is an essential part of our diet. By essential, I mean that you can't live without glucose. While a sugar-free diet sounds like a healthy thing, it can actually be deadly.

If you eliminate sugar from your diet, your cells would get their energy from other sources, like breaking down fat or from your own body tissue. This releases adrenaline and cortisol, the same hormones released during our body's fight or flight response. When people turn to a sugar-free die, they feel good at first because of these hormones. However, our bodies aren't meant to live off of adrenaline and cortisol.

Eliminating sugar can destroy metabolism, lead to a weakened immune system, poor digestion, impaired sexual function, and accelerate aging. Without enough sugar, your body would fail. Your brain needs glucose to function. If you don't have enough sugar in your bloodstream, you would get dizzy, faint, and possibly go into a coma or even die.

Clearly the body needs sugar to live. But let's take a look at the other benefits of sugar:

ENERGY SOURCE
Glucose from sugar is the body's preferred and most efficient source of energy. Unless you want to sit around reading all day, you're going to need energy to get off your rear end and do something. Sugar can be that kick in the pants you need.

HEALTHY SKIN
Sugar contains glycolic acid which helps maintain healthy skin. We all know acid is good for your skin.

HELPS US EAT OTHER HEALTHFUL FOODS
Even the American Heart Association acknowledges the health benefit of sugar in the diet, saying "In fact, when sugars are added to otherwise nutrient rich foods, such sugar-sweetened dairy products like flavored milk and yogurt and sugar-sweetened cereals, the quality of children's and adolescents' diets improved, and in case of flavored milks, no adverse effects on weight status were found." Translation: sugar makes stuff taste good and doesn't make you fat.

NATURAL
Sugar is a natural and less processed food than other sweeteners like high-fructose corn syrup. If you need to sweeten your food, don't mess around with artificial sweeteners, use the real stuff. Plain old sugar.

ENVIRONMENTAL BENEFITS
Sugar is made from the plants sugar cane and sugar beets, which are renewable natural resources. Sugar is environmentally friendly as it's produced without pesticides and other harmful products. This could be important to you if you're the tree-hugging hippy type.

CARBS
The partner in crime to sugar is carbs. Carbs are also feared and hated.

What is a carb? Carbohydrates are in all kinds of foods from breads and pastas to fruits and vegetables. Our bodies break carbs down into glucose or sugars that we use for energy. Carbs are the main source of energy for the body. Carbs are needed by every vital organ in our body, including the brain, heart, and liver. Carbs also helps with muscle function, growth, and regulation of body temperature.

LOW CARB DIETS

In the 1990's low carb diets, like the Adkins Diet, became popular. I know low carb diets are all the craze, but they go against the grain. Eliminating carbs is a bad idea and causes all kinds of health ramifications.

People on low-carb diets can lose significant weight quickly. However, they also regained more weight back in the long run. A study published in the New England Journal of Medicine showed that low-carb dieters initially lost more weight than low-fat dieters, but in the second half of the year the weight came back.

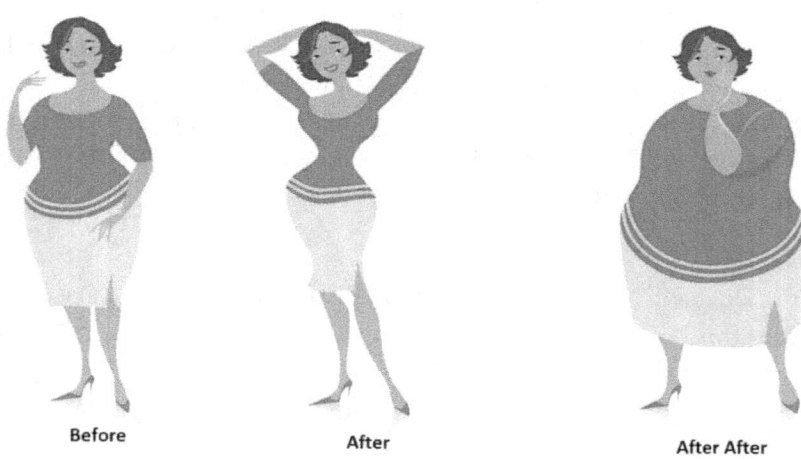

Before   After   After After

When you drop your carb consumption low enough, your body eventually begins to burn muscle and fat which may sound good, but it also comes with complications like being tired, lightheaded, nauseated, headaches, trouble concentrating, and bad breath. That's enough side effects to make it sound like a prescription drug commercial.

The loss of muscle also harms your health as your metabolism will slow. Muscle burns more calories, and with less of it, you'll burn less calories.

Low carb diets may also be worse for your insulin sensitivity. Your body needs a certain amount of carbs for the pancreas to function properly.

Eliminating carbs is a bad idea and bad for your health. So should we eat carbs? Yes! I know people avoid carbs because they think eating carbs makes them fat. This is simply not true. Let's look at the people in the world that consume a large amount of carbs. Asians eat tons of rice. They aren't fat. French people eat white bread. The French aren't fat. Italians eat semolina pasta. The Italians don't have the obesity problem as America does. Eating a lot of carbs, even white bread and pasta, doesn't make you fat.

Let's end the chapter with a joke. Have you heard about the pasta diet?

It has a few simple steps:

1. You walk pasta da bakery.
2. You walk pasta da candy store.
3. You walk pasta da ice cream shop.
4. You walk pasta da table and da fridge.

It's similar to another joke.

You have many weight loss options:

1. Gastric bypass
2. Donut bypass
3. Pizza bypass
4. Buffet bypass

FAKE TESTIMONIAL #3

LIZ ONNIA: **I FELT LIKE I DIDN'T GAIN ANY WEIGHT WHILE I WAS "PREGNANT"**

I was working at a local donut shop. I know, working at a donut shop seems like it would be a diet disaster. Honestly, I didn't eat the donuts. I saw how they were made. And, I only weighed 135 pounds so I didn't think I had a weight issue. I didn't have a problem selling dozens of donuts all night

One day I saw one of our regulars reading a book as he sat in the shop eating a box of donuts. I asked him what he was reading. He said it was a new book called the Contrarian Diet. He explained that's why he ordered a dozen donuts that day instead of his normal two donuts. He started the new diet because on one hand he wanted to lose weight, but on the other hand he wanted a donut. He compromised and found a diet that allowed him to eat donuts. He explained to me that the Contrarian Diet promoted a diet rich in sugar, carbs, sodium, and fat. You could eat anything you want and not exercise.

I was intrigued. That didn't sound like a diet. That sounded too good to be true. When I got home, I ordered a copy of the Contrarian Diet online. I stayed up all night reading it (I'm a slow reader).

I had never been on a diet before. I just tried to eat small portions, eat a lot of salad, and pass up deserts. I wasn't exactly skinny, but I wasn't fat either. The Contrarian Diet actually sounded fun. I loved Italian food, but I usually tried to limit myself. If I started the Contrarian Diet at least I'd have a good excuse for going hog wild eating pasta. I'd just tell people I'm on the Contrarian Diet when they ask why I'm eating like a pig.

I started the Contrarian Diet and ate plates and plates of pasta. I had spaghetti alla carbonara, puttanesca, fettuccine alfredo, baked rotini, three cheese lasagna, penne with vodka sauce, ricotta gnocchi, ravioli with pesto, and of course my favorite Spaghetti O's with meatballs!

Pretty soon people starting asking me when I was due or if I was having a baby boy or girl. I would say, "No, I'm not pregnant. I'm just on the Contrarian Diet." At first I was a little confused why people assumed I was pregnant. I didn't feel like I gained any weight. When I looked in the mirror, I didn't think I was heavier. Maybe it was because I look in the mirror every day and the change was so gradual I didn't notice. I tried the bathroom scale. Somehow I gained 20 pounds.

I wasn't sure if I should continue the Contrarian Diet or not. On one hand, I really enjoyed eating whatever I wanted. But on the other hand, it was going to get expensive buying new clothes. Luckily, a friend of mine that assumed I was pregnant gave me a bunch of her hand-me-down maternity clothes.

Having everyone assume you're pregnant wasn't necessarily a bad thing. People would hold the door open for me, cars would immediately stop when I was crossing the street, people would give up their seat for me when I got on the bus, I could park closer at the store, and it made for a good excuse when I didn't want to do something. I even had a couple friends buy me baby shower gifts.

I wasn't pregnant, but I just kind of played along. I'm not quite sure what I'm going to do once the nine months go by, but in the meantime I'm loving my new diet and the perks of being pregnant with my food baby. I'm also taking advantage of my employee discount at the donut shop. Thank you Contrarian Diet for changing my life!

Chapter 4

SODIUM IS SODIUM GOOD

". . .all of us have in our veins the exact same percentage of salt in our blood that exists in the ocean, and, therefore, we have salt in our blood, in our sweat, in our tears. We are tied to the ocean. And, when we go back to the sea. . . we are going back to whence we came." - John F. Kennedy

"I always take life with a grain of salt. . . plus a slice of lemon. . . and a shot of tequila." – Unknown

Salt is the second evil food in the eyes of the public. Like our friends sugar and carbs in the last chapter, salt has become feared and hated by people.

The fear mongers have told us that we need to cut back on salt in order to lower our risk of heart disease and stroke. Despite any scientific proof that a low sodium diet reduces heart disease, we've all been convinced that salt is bad for us. Up until the 1970's, the only ones on earth that hated salt were slugs. Now everyone hates salt.

People no longer salt their food at meal times. The salt shaker is on the verge of extinction, and soon will go the way of the ash tray. People who salt their food are viewed the same way as people who drive while texting. It's viewed as irresponsible and risky. If you do attempt to salt your food, your fellow diners will inform you of your social faux pas through dirty looks and snide comments.

For thousands and thousands of years, people actually loved salt. Throughout human history, salt has been a desirable and valuable commodity. People discovered the importance of salt long before recorded history. Salt has been used as a preservative for food, a way to enhance the taste of food, and as a vicious weapon to rub into our enemies' wounds. Salt continues to this day to be one of the most effective and widely used preservatives for food.

Salt has been valued so much that is has been used as money. People used to refer to salt as white gold. The word "salary" is derived from salt as Roman soldiers were paid in salt. In ancient Greece, salt was traded for slaves, which created the expression, "not worth his salt." Even up until the 20th century, salt bars were used as money in parts of Ethiopia.

Why after thousands of years did salt go from being a valuable commodity referred to as white gold to becoming an evil white powder on par with sugar?

The same decade disco became cool is the same decade that salt became not-cool. In hind sight, maybe we had it backwards.

HEALTH BENEFITS OF SALT
We have been told that salt is bad for our diet. This simply isn't true. Let's shake things up a bit by looking at the health benefits of salt.

Salt is an essential part of your diet. By essential, I mean you need it to live. Just like sugar, if you completely eliminate salt from your diet, you'll fall over dead. Every cell in your body contains salt. Human blood contains 0.9% salt. While salt and sodium aren't the same thing, sodium is the main component of salt (salt's chemical name is sodium chloride). People, animals, and even many plants need salt to live. If you don't get enough salt, you'll die. In fact, every year a few marathon runners die from hyponatremia as they deplete themselves of salt.

Other than keeping you alive, here's a brief list of the other ways salt helps your body:

- Helps maintain muscle tone and strength. That's why Popeye ate canned spinach instead of fresh spinach. It was the sodium in the can that made him strong, not the spinach.
- Eliminates persistent dry coughs. Rather than stop smoking, just increase your salt intake.
- Keeps your heartbeat steady. I hear that's important.
- It's a strong anti-stress element for the body. That's why bars serve both alcohol and salty nuts. They're both use for medicinal purposes to relieve stress.

- Regulates blood pressure and blood volume, and controls blood sugar levels. These are all important if you have a friend that's a vampire.
- It's a natural antihistamine. Which I guess counteracts pepper's ability to make us sneeze.
- Clears up congestion in the sinuses. If salt doesn't work, try Chinese mustard.
- Clears mucus plugs and sticky phlegm in the lungs, particularly in asthma and cystic fibrosis. You may think it's mucus and phlegm, but it's not.
- Lowers adrenaline spikes. As a Contrarian dieter, you don't need adrenaline since you're lazy.
- Prevents gout and gouty arthritis. So does cherry juice, but salt tastes better on steak and eggs.
- Helps treat emotional disorders. So does ice cream.
- Stops excess saliva production. Just in case you drool too much.
- Strengthens bone structure. Osteoporosis, in many ways, is a result of salt and water shortage in the body. Got salt?
- It's a natural hypnotic. Now I'm going to count backwards from ten and after I do you're going to get sleepy and then write a positive review about this book.
- Is a four lettered word you can say without getting your mouth washed out with soap.
- Encourages a healthy weight and fast metabolism. Sounds like a natural diet pill to me.
- Can combat hypothermia. Next time your boat hits an iceberg, just drink the freezing ocean water to stay warm.
- Helps kidneys pass excess acidity into the urine. So basically, you're able to pee acid. That could be painful.
- Generates hydroelectric energy in your body's cells. Damn!
- Provides your body with all essential mineral and every necessary trace mineral it needs to thrive. That makes burgers and fries health food.
- Helps maintain sexuality and libido. That's why I keep a salt shaker on my night stand.

After reading all of the health benefits of salt, maybe you won't feel so guilty next time you order a large tub of popcorn at the movies or eat all of the pub mix at the bar while waiting for your beer.

LOW-SALT DIET IS BAD

We've been lead to believe that salt is bad for us and that we should cut down on our salt intake. We've been told the less salt we eat, the better. However, this is completely wrong.

One of the biggest surprises about the Contrarian Diet is that a low sodium diet can increase your risk of heart disease, stroke, and even death. Take those low-sodium diets with a grain of salt. I understand that you may not trust the health advice in this book, but consider these headlines from very reliable sources:

"Low-Salt Diets May Pose Health Risks, Study Finds." - The Wall Street Journal, August 14, 2014

"No Benefit Seen in Sharp Limits on Salt in Diet." - The New York Times, May 14, 2013

"Salt, Healthy? Why It Might No Longer Be Public Enemy No. 1." - Reader's Digest

"Salt is Good for You." – German Pretzel Factory Employee Newsletter

---

The Food and Drug Administration recommends limiting our sodium to 2,300 milligrams a day. The American Heart Association suggests an even lower limit of just 1,500 milligrams a day. Yet, cutting back on salt hasn't been shown to result in any health benefit. On the contrary, low salt diets have been shown to increase your risk of death.

There are hundreds of studies on the effects of sodium on diet. The simple fact is that these studies show more evidence that salt is good for you.

There is no scientific proof that a low salt diet is good for you. Rather, there is a lot of evidence that a low sodium diet is harmful.

For people with high blood pressure, lowering salt may reduce blood pressure. However, most of us don't have high blood pressure, only 1 in 3 people do. That doesn't seem to matter, because doctors and nutritionists tells us everyone in the entire country needs to be on a low-sodium diet.

Even for people with high blood pressure, a low sodium diet may do more harm than good. A study by Copenhagen University Hospital showed that a low sodium diet did reduce blood pressure by 3.5% for people with hypertension. However, it also raised their triglycerides and cholesterol. Additionally, it boosted their levels of aldosterone and norepinephrine, two hormones that can increase insulin resistance over time.

A Canadian study showed that reducing sodium intake to less than 3,000 milligrams a day, which both the FDA and American Heart Association recommend you do, results in a 27% higher risk of death or serious cardiovascular event within four years.

Another study based on people from New York City found that people on low sodium diets had more than four times as many heart attacks as those on normal sodium diets. If you live in New York, it sounds like it may be a good idea to eat more salt.

How Much Salt is Safe to Eat?
Everyone's need will vary depending on their age, gender, genetics, and lifestyle. Listen to your body. Let your salt craving dictate how much salt to eat. Americans consume about 3,500 milligrams of salt a day, with men consuming more than women. Studies show that most people can tolerate a wide range of sodium consumption, ranging from 250 milligrams to over 30,000 milligrams a day.

Researchers have recently suggested the safest range may be between 2,645 to 4,945 milligrams a day. That's over three times the level of sodium that the American Heart Association is trying to limit us to.

FAKE TESTIMONIAL #4

MEGAN BACON: **I HAVEN'T LOST ANY WEIGHT, BUT I HAVE LOST MY HUSBAND**

All my life I've been a little overweight. I'm not fat, but I do weigh 400 pounds because I'm big boned. I've always wanted to be skinny like the girls in the magazines and on TV, because everyone knows being skinny makes you happy.

I've been on all the fad diets and none of them work. I gained 20 pounds on Jenny Craig, 50 pounds on Atkins, 10 pounds on Weight Watchers, and 120 pounds on Paleo (I ate a small dinosaur). Diets just make you fat.

So one day I made a doctor appointment to discuss weight loss. I told her I didn't want another fad diet because I've been on every fad diet and they simply don't work. I also didn't want surgery because my Aunt Mildred died during liposuction surgery, and that really sucked.

My doctor recommended the Contrarian Diet. Hey, physician assisted suicide is legal in my state – what do you expect? So I tried the Contrarian Diet. So far, I haven't lost any weight, but I do have to say that this is the easiest diet ever. I've been on diets that restricted salt and I craved it so much. Low or no salt foods are not only hard to find, but they have no taste. No salt soup is like drinking canned water. And Mrs. Dash… I just wanted to dash her to pieces. The low / no salt diet is just torture. The fact that the Contrarian Diet not only allows salty food, but encourages a diet rich is sodium is one of the main reasons I love the Contrarian Diet so far.

It's only been two months on the Contrarian Diet so far for me. But already I can taste a difference. My food tastes so much better. I've reintroduced a lot of stuff back into my eating, like popcorn, chips, pretzels, burgers, fries, tots, peanuts (they put the nut into nutrition), and beef jerky. I find myself salting things all the time now too. Not just meat and potatoes, but also things like pizza, and sometimes I just tilt my head back and shake a little salt right on my tongue. My favorite food is pizza with pepperoni and bacon. I love to salt my pizza. It makes the greasy pepperoni and bacon bits taste so much better.

To be honest, I did gain a few pounds when I started the Contrarian Diet, but only 40 or 50. My husband started lecturing me about what I was eating, so I ate him too. No, he didn't taste like chicken. But I did need quite a bit of salt to make it palatable.

Now I'm single, but I don't mind because that leaves more food for me. I don't really care because I love this diet. We've all heard that weight loss is a journey, not a race. I don't expect to slim down overnight. But I am going to enjoy all the fine salty foods as I do. I really expect this to change my life. I don't want to see another disgusting salad again or go on another yo yo diet. This diet is sodium easy, and I'm sticking to it. Of course, I stick to almost everything now that I'm eating this much sodium.

Chapter 5

GOOD FATS, THERE ARE NO BAD FATS

"No diet will remove all the fat from your body because the brain is entirely fat. Without a brain, you might look good, but all you could do is run for public office." - George Bernard Shaw

"McDonalds will always have a place in my heart...where the fat will build up in my valves and eventually kill me." - Unknown

Fat is the third and final evil food group, along with sugar/carbs and salt.

Dieters tend to be fat-a-phobes. We've all known that health nut that gets up the morning and eats a non-fat yogurt and a banana for breakfast. At lunch, they order their salad with the dressing "on the side." For dinner, they steam their vegetables.

They make snide comments to people eating real food like "That's a coronary episode on a plate," or "Can I have a heart attack with that burger, please?"

Where did this idea of fat being bad for you ever come from? Were the researchers on drugs when they came up with that hypothesis?

Actually, they were. Back in the 60's a bunch of bell-bottom pants, tie-dye shirt wearing scientists with long hair and high on drugs decided that fat was bad. They came up with the idea that saturated fat raised bad cholesterol in the blood and lead to heart disease. This crazy idea lead to the hugely popular low-fat diet. In the 1980's we were taught to hate fat as the fat-free craze swept the nation.

The idea behind the low-fat craze is that fat has nine calories per gram, while carbs and protein only have four calories per gram. The idea is that if you cut out fat, you'll eat less calories and in turn lose weight.

Needless to say, the low-fat diet craze wasn't successful. Actually, the rate of obesity increased with the start of the low-fat diet as shown in the chart below.

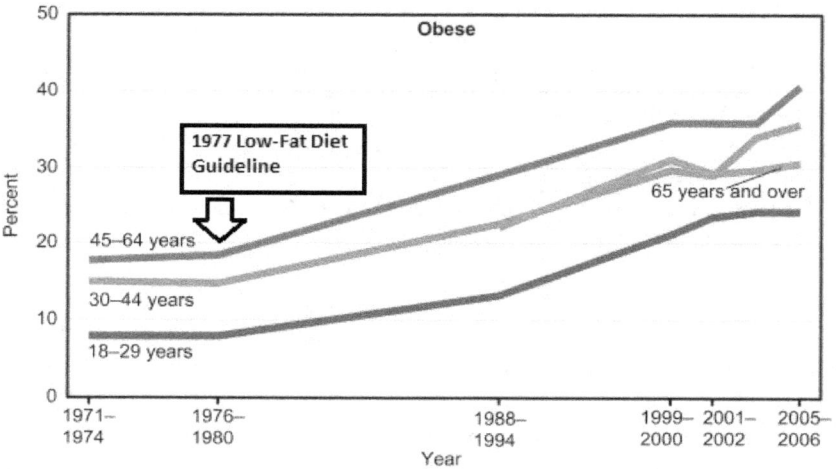

Source: National Center for Health Statistics. Health, United States, 2008: With Special Feature on the Health of Young Adults.

While the low-fat diet sounded logical to a bunch of hippy researchers that decided to switch from eating high-fat magical brownies to the lower fat choice of psychedelic mushrooms, in reality it simply didn't work. Low-fat food is less fulfilling than high fat foods and you simply eat more low-fat foods. Sometimes a lot more.

WHAT IS FAT?
Fat is an essential nutrient. An essential nutrient, as pointed out in the last couple chapters, is something necessary for life. Just like sugar and salt, if you don't eat fat you'll die. Even the USDA admits that some amount of saturated fat is necessary for life.

Fat is found in oils, butters, nuts, fatty fish, meats, dairy, and some foods like avocados and chocolate cake. You can even find fat in pizza, ice cream, and candy bars.

HEALTH BENEFITS OF FAT

40

Here are some of the health benefits of fat:

Fat supplies our bodies with energy. This is why overweight people make great long distance runners.

Some fats can help prevent certain cancers, aid in weight loss, and help your body absorb nutrients more effectively. Keep that in mind next time you're ordering food at the drive thru.

Fat can help you feel full, so you eat less overall. Like after you eat a dozen donuts. You feel so full you can't eat another bite of anything.

Fat helps with the absorption of certain vitamins and phytonutrients, which are compounds in plants that are thought to promote health. Way to go fat!

Fat improves dietary adherence. You'll stick to a diet better if you like its taste. Meals with some fats are tastier. That's why people spread peanut butter on celery. It makes something disgusting somewhat tolerable. Who am I kidding? We all just lick off the peanut butter and throw away the celery.

Like our friends sugar and salt, there is a lot of misunderstandings and misinformation about fat. Let's debunk a couple of the big fat myths:

BIG FAT MYTH #1. FAT MAKES YOU FAT

Not true. The Harvard School of Public Health titles their page on fats with, "It's time to End the Low-Fat Myth." I didn't bother reading anything else on the page, but I think their title sums it up nicely. Eating fat doesn't make you fat. Eating or drinking more calories than you need from any source, whether it's fat, carbs, protein, or alcohol can lead to weight gain.

Carefully-conducted clinical trials find that following a low-fat diet doesn't make it easier to lose weight or keep it off. In fact, volunteers who follow moderate or high-fat diets lose just as much weight, and in some studies a bit more, as those who follow low-fat diets.

If eating fat makes you fat, explain French people to me. The French eat croissants, cheese, ratatouille, French fries, French toast, French vanilla ice cream, and yet they aren't fat.

Big Fat Myth #2. Fat Causes Heart Disease

Cardiologists have spread the myth that high cholesterol causes heart disease. However, there are many studies that contradict this idea.

A 2012 Norwegian University of Science and Technology study examined the health and lifestyle habits of more than 52,000 people and found that women with high cholesterol had a 28 percent lower mortality risk than women with low cholesterol.

In the British Medical Journal in 2013, a cardiologist named Aseem Malhotra argued that lowering your saturated fat consumption, as most physicians recommend, actually contributes to making you fat and increasing your risk of heart disease.

The Annals of Internal Medicine in March 2014, using data compiled from nearly 80 studies and more than a half million people, found that people who consume higher amounts of saturated fat have no more heart disease than those who consume less.

If eating a high fat diet leads to heart disease and premature death, then how to you explain the 105-year-old Texan woman who claimed eating bacon lead to her long life. Pearl Cantrell told NBC affiliate KRBC when asked her secret to living so long, "I love bacon. I eat it every day." Of course when Oscar Mayer caught wind of what she said, they sent the Wienermobile to her house with a gift of free bacon. I don't know what's more exciting. Living to be 105 years old, or having the Weinermobile show up at your house.

That reminds me of a joke.

The French eat a lot fat and suffer fewer heart attacks than Americans.

The Japanese eat very little fat and suffer fewer heart attacks than Americans.

The Chinese drink very little red wine and suffer fewer heart attacks than Americans.

The Italians drink a lot of red wine and suffer fewer heart attacks than Americans.

42

The Germans drink a lot of beer and eat a lot of sausage and fat and suffer fewer heart attacks than Americans.

Conclusion: Eat and drink what you like, as speaking English is apparently what kills you.

FAKE TESTIMONIAL #5
PETER PANTS: **I WENT ON THE CONTRARIAN DIET AND I'M OFF MY MEDS**

Back in my day, when I was a young whippersnapper, I used to be skinny. I walked 12 miles up hill in the snow just to get to school. That was each way. I don't know how it was uphill each way, but it was.

These days I just sit at home in my rocking chair reading the newspaper and trying to remember what day it is. Usually I start out the day taking my pills and then reading the obituaries to find any eligible women. Then I take a nap. When I wake up, I feel like a newborn baby. No hair, no teeth, and I wet my pants.

A few years back, I gained a little weight. I had decided to eat like crazy in order to fill out my wrinkles. It didn't work. I did gain weight, but I still have all my wrinkles.

I'm only 82, and I want to get back into shape before I get too old. I'm 5'6" and weigh 220 pounds. According to the BMI chart, I'm too short.

I recently went to the doctor and he said I needed to lose some weight. I told him that I'm too old to jog, bike, or swim. The doc told me I just needed to do anything that would keep me active.

I started playing games at the Senior Center, like sag you're it, hide and pee, musical recliners, and kick the bucket. None of those games worked. I didn't lose any weight.

I knew I needed to do something more drastic. I had heard about the Contrarian Diet on one of those late night infomercials on TV that targets vulnerable seniors like me. So I ordered the book and read it.

The Contrarian Diet fits my lifestyle. I can sit at home in my rocking chair eating cookies, donuts, and pie. I can't remember what I weighed before starting the Contrarian Diet, or even what pills I'm supposed to take, but I don't really care anymore. It's nice being able to eat fatty foods, feel good, not exercise, and be off my meds.

Chapter 6

ICE CREAM, AM I FAT YET?

"Never trust a skinny ice cream man." - BEN COHEN

"You can't buy happiness but you can buy ice cream and that's kind of the same thing."
- Unknown

Like any food that combines high levels of sugar and fat, ice cream tastes yummy!

The average American eats almost five gallons a year. Some Americans, like the readers of this book, eat five gallons a month. Whether you eat ice cream in moderation or like a pig at a feeding trough, everyone loves ice cream. Despite our love of ice cream, most people feel guilty about eating it. They've bought into the lie that ice cream is bad.

The truth is ice cream is good for you! Ice cream is made of natural, healthful ingredients like milk, cream, sugar, and flavoring. In the preceding chapters we've already discovered that fats and sugars are good. Ice cream is made up of these good ingredients.

It doesn't matter if you like chocolate or vanilla, one scoop or two, or plain cones, sugar cones, waffle cones, or pine cones. It's all good.

Unfortunately, ice cream has been labelled as junk food. Anyone that claims that ice cream is an important and healthful addition to your diet would be ridiculed. Reality, however, is ice cream has several health benefits. If you're thinking eating ice cream for nutritional value is just a joke, you're mistaken. There really is research that supports the health benefits of ice cream. Here's the scoop:

HEALTH BENEFITS OF ICE CREAM

Before we get into the health benefits of ice cream, let's talk about serving size. If you just look at the nutritional information on a carton of ice cream,

45

it may seem like ice cream doesn't have a very large percentage of vitamins and minerals. This is mainly due to the serving size. If you look carefully at the nutritional information, it claims that a serving size of ice cream is only ½ cup. Who eats only ½ cup of ice cream? I normally put at least 2 cups of ice cream in my first bowl of ice cream, so it's more accurate to quadruple all of the nutritional information. For the purposes below, a serving of ice cream is equal to 2 cups.

CALCIUM

Ice cream is a dairy product, which is one of the four food groups if I'm not mistaken. As a dairy product, ice cream is high in calcium which helps build strong and healthy bones. A single serving of ice cream provides 40% of the recommended daily calcium allowance. Because of its high calcium content, ice cream can also help reduce the risk of osteoporosis. Calcium does good things for your body, and ice cream is probably the most delicious source of calcium available.

PHOSPHORUS

Ice cream also contains a good amount of phosphorus. A single serving provides about 40% of the recommended dietary allowance for phosphorus. Phosphorus helps in the formation of bones and teeth. Without phosphorus you would look like a toothless Jabba the Hut.

POTASSIUM

Bananas aren't the only source of potassium. While most people get their potassium from fruits and veggies, another source for potassium is ice cream! The potassium in ice cream can help lower your blood pressure. I've actually blown off taking blood pressure pills and just eat ice cream instead.

PROTEIN

Ice cream has about 8 grams of protein per serving. Protein is important in building and repairing skin. Since the body doesn't store protein, food with protein, like ice cream, is important to eat on a regular basis.

VITAMIN A

Ice cream contains Vitamin A. There's no need to eat carrots. Just grab a bowl or two of ice cream. Vitamin A helps you see in low light and see colors. Vitamin A is important in helping you find your way through the dark into the kitchen at night and find the right flavor ice cream in the freezer.

B VITAMINS

Ice cream contains Thiamin (Vitamin B1), Riboflavin (Vitamin B2), Niacin (Vitamin B3), Vitamin B-6, Vitamin B-12, and Folic Acid. While they sound like Bingo numbers, they actually are important for energy metabolism, breaking down fats, proteins, and carbohydrates in the body.

VITAMIN C

A serving of ice cream has about 16% of the recommended dietary allowance for vitamin C. You can increase this significantly by making ice cream floats out of orange juice. Vitamin C is a powerful antioxidant that prevents scurvy. If you're a pirate or sailor, you may want to eat a lot of ice cream when you're in port. Besides preventing scurvy, Vitamin C also helps protect against many types of cancers, immune system deficiencies, cardiovascular disease, prenatal problems, cataracts, and skin wrinkling.

VITAMIN D

Vitamin D helps your body absorb calcium. Two fun ways to get Vitamin D are eating ice cream (of course) and sun tanning. Neither one poses any sort of health risk as far as I'm aware. Although, I am banned from practicing medicine by the Medical Board in all 50 states.

VITAMIN E

Vitamin E is an antioxidant. You can get Vitamin E from things like vegetable oil, nuts, seeds, and leafy greens. But why do that when you can eat ice cream?

VITAMIN K

Ice cream contains Vitamin K, which helps with blood clotting. This is important in case you injure yourself with your spoon while eating ice cream. While ice cream isn't very high in Vitamin K, if you eat ice cream in large amounts you will get a significant source.

ENERGY

Ice cream is also a great source of energy. It's rich with carbohydrates, fats, and proteins, which are all needed for our bodies to produce energy.

Energy is important as that's how you're able to lift your body off the couch, stagger to the kitchen, open the refrigerator door, and scoop yourself a couple bowls of ice cream. Without energy, you couldn't eat ice cream.

FERTILITY

Ice cream may also help with fertility. A Harvard study suggests that alcohol isn't the only thing that can lead to pregnancy, so can ice cream. The study published in the journal Human Reproduction suggests that consuming full-fat milk or ice cream may improve your chances of getting pregnant. Women who ate ice cream two or more times a week had a 38% lower risk of ovulation-related infertility than women who didn't eat as much ice cream.

STRESS RELIEVER

You may have already discovered this on your own, but ice cream is a stress reliever. Eating ice cream stimulates the thrombotonin, which helps with happiness and stress relief. Ice cream contains L-triptophane (same as Thanksgiving turkey), a natural tranquilizer that also helps in relaxing the nervous system.

ICE CREAM MAY HELP YOU LOSE WEIGHT

Avoiding ice cream may not help you get skinny. Eating ice cream may help you lose weight. A study published in the American Journal of Clinical Nutrition found that women who ate at least one daily serving of full-fat dairy products, such as ice cream, gained less weight than those who didn't.

Apparently the calcium in ice cream is the key to the weight loss. If you don't get enough calcium your body triggers fat cells to store fat and get bigger. Also ice cream is more satisfying than veggies, so dieters don't go on eating binges.

There is even a diet that revolves around eating ice cream to lose weight. Holly McCord, a nutrition editor for Prevention magazine and a registered dietitian, has a book called The Ice Cream Diet. She shows research that supports eating high calcium foods like ice cream to lose weight, reduce PMS, reduce the risk of colon cancer, and lower blood pressure.

THE DANGER OF ICE CREAM

Of course, it wouldn't be responsible to recommend a diet of ice cream without the obvious danger to your health of eating too much ice cream.

While many people eat ice cream without thinking of the health consequences, eating too much ice cream can have a major effect on your health. You could develop sphenopalatine ganglioneuralgia.

The main symptom of sphenopalatine ganglioneuralgia is excruciating pain in the midfrontal area of the head. People who suffer from sphenopalatine ganglioneuralgia experience the same pain produced when doctors drill into the inner table of the skull in patients that are awake.

The sharp, stabbing pain caused by sphenopalatine ganglioneuralgia increases and peaks in intensity after 30 to 60 seconds. The pain can last up to five minutes, and occasionally even longer.

The pain can also be located in the temporal or retro-orbital region (behind the eye). It can also be accompanied by a toothache.

The pain is so intense that people suffering from sphenopalatine ganglioneuralgia will grab their head and yell.

Sphenopalatine ganglioneuralgia happens when something very cold touches the upper-palate (roof of the mouth). It tends to occur when the weather is hot and the victim is consuming something cold too quickly. Common terms for this serious condition are "ice cream headache" or simply "brain freeze."

While eating ice cream is almost always an enjoyable experience, the reader is highly cautioned about the real risk of sphenopalatine ganglioneuralgia.

The best cure for ice cream headache, however, is prevention. You can take a couple simple steps to safer ice cream eating. First, eat slower. Second, try to avoid placing ice cream on the back of the palate (roof of the mouth).

If you find yourself an unfortunate victim of ice cream headache, here are some techniques used by actually survivors that may lower the pain and duration of the attack.

Some people claim that pressing your tongue against the roof of the mouth with help. Others suggest drinking something warm (at least warmer than the ice cream). Still others have used an ancient Yoga anti-ice cream headache breathing technique that involves breathing in through the mouth and out through the nose. The key to all of these techniques is to somehow warm the area that is causing the brain freeze.

FAKE TESTIMONIAL #6
ROCKY RHODE: **I MADE A NEW YEAR'S RESOLUTION TO LOSE 20 POUNDS**

I'm not fat or anything, but I do eat ice cream a lot more than most people. I have my alarm clock set up with the song the ice cream man plays so that I can wake up happy and ready to eat ice cream. I also live in San Antonio, so I like driving around town yelling, "Remember the Al La Mode!"

I routinely eat ice cream for breakfast. People think that eating ice cream for breakfast is strange, but it's not that different than eating a bowl of cereal. Think about it. If you pour yourself a bowl of sugary cereal and top it with milk, you're pretty much eating sugar and fat for breakfast. That's all ice cream is. A frozen bowl of cereal.

For lunch I normally have an ice cream sandwich. In the evening, I have a light dinner like a bowl of ice cream and an ice cream bar for dessert.

Even though I wasn't eating a lot, I had noticed that I was gaining a lot of weight. I told myself that I was going to go on a diet, so I did a ton of research to find a diet compatible with what I love to eat. I came across the Contrarian Diet.

At first I was confused because I was pretty much eating ice cream for three meals a day. I shouldn't be gaining weight. Ice cream is good for you. Then I looked into what kinds of ice cream I was eating: Strawberry, Raspberry Swirl, Orange Pineapple, Apple Cinnamon Gelato, Spumoni, Banana Nut, Green Tea, Apple Walnut, Black Cherry, Orange Sherbet, Lemon Lime Sorbet, Mango Sorbet, Peaches n' Cream, and other fruity ice cream flavors that I thought were healthful.

It turned out that it wasn't the ice cream that was making me gain weight. It was the type of ice cream I was eating. When I got rid of the fruity ice cream flavors and switched to ice cream flavors that had more fatty, sugary goodness in them, I felt so much better. Now I eat flavors like: Butter Chocolate Chip, Mud Pie, Cotton Candy Twist, Peppermint Candy, Candy Bar Blast, Moose Tracks, Cookie Dough, Butterscotch Swirl, Kahlua Almond Fudge, Espresso Fudge Chip, Chocolate Fudge, Peanut Butter Fudge Swirl, Chocolate Marshmallow, Double Chocolate Brownie, Mint Chocolate Cookie, and Rocky Road.

I'm so glad I discovered the Contrarian Diet. I would have gone on eating all of the wrong flavors of ice cream without this diet. The Contrarian Diet has definitely been a life changer. I feel so much better now. I had made a New Year's resolution to lose 20 pounds, and I only have 30 more pounds to go.

Chapter 7

PIZZA, IS IT HEART DISEASE YET?

"You better cut the pizza in four pieces because I'm not hungry enough to eat six." - *Yogi Berra*

"My diet has me avoiding all fried foods... which is why I'm so happy that pizza is baked!" - *Unknown*

Pizza may be the only food that contains all four food groups, tastes good, and can be delivered to your house in under 30 minutes.

Maybe that's why pizza is the most popular meal in the entire world. Every day more than 40 million Americans eat pizza. Every year, Americans eat over 23 pounds of pizza.

Let's take a quick trip back in time and see how pizza originated.

A BRIEF HISTORY OF PIZZA
Pizza wasn't exactly born. It's more accurate to say pizza evolved over time.

The story of pizza begins in prehistoric times. Since by definition prehistoric means there's no record of it, we can only guess how it was made. Soon after fire was invented, cavemen likely built wood fired brick ovens out of large stones to bake flatbread with toppings. Woolly Mammoth with pineapple was probably a tribe favorite. After the invention of the wheel, it was likely that you could have one of these flatbreads with toppings delivered to your cave in 30 minutes or less.

These early forms of pizza likely gave birth to civilization. As the cavemen ate these flatbread pizzas, they became so fat and lazy that they almost completely gave up on hunting and gathering. They started farming in order to grow more ingredients to make dough for their flatbreads. Soon cities popped up, thanks to pizza.

History books tell us that people continued to eat flatbread with toppings. The ancient Greeks topped their flatbread with oils, olives, and dates (large raisins, not their girlfriends). In the 6th century B.C, the soldiers of Darius the Great made a type of red neck version of pizza by baking flat bread on their shields and covering it with cheese and dates (these may have been their girlfriends… they were rednecks). Evidence of early pizza making has even been uncovered in Pompeii that shows the people there made and ate an early version of pizza, a flatbread topped with lava and ash.

The modern pizza didn't take shape until later. In 1522, Christopher Columbus sailed the ocean blue. I know he sailed the ocean blue in 1492, but something more important happened in 1522 when he once again sailed the ocean blue. 1522 was the year that the tomato was imported from South America to Europe. That meant no more eating crappy flatbread topped with dates.

Southern Italy was a great place to grow tomatoes. After people got over the fear of tomatoes as they thought tomatoes were poisonous, they began eating them and they became a popular food in the 1600's. Of course wearing lace collars and broad funny hats were popular at that time too.

Around the same time, mozzarella cheese began to catch on. The Italians made mozzarella from water buffalo milk, called mozzarella di bufla. The introduction of the tomato to Italy and the popularity of mozzarella cheese helped the evolution of pizza. However, the modern pizza wasn't developed until the 1800's.

Like pizza itself, the word "pizza" has evolved overtime. The word is believed to come from the Old Italian word "pizziare" which means "a point", which makes sense since a slice of pizza is triangular in shape and has a point on the end. Later it became "pizzicare" which means to pinch, or to pluck, which makes no sense unless the Italians were drunk at the time they came up with this term. By the 1800's the word pizza was commonly used.

Naples, Italy is where modern pizza was developed. Naples was a waterfront city. It also had a large population of poor people, who spent most of their time outdoors. The flat bread covered in tomatoes and cheese made for a cheap meal that could be carried away and eaten. It could be eaten for breakfast, lunch, and dinner. Pizza was sold on the streets, and eventually in restaurants. Pizzeri Brandi is allegedly the first pizzeria in Naples. It opened in 1780 and is still selling pizza today.

In 1889, King Umberto I and Queen Margherita visited Naples and decided to slum it and try the local pizza. The story goes that the owner of Pizzeria Brandi, Raffaele Esposito, made them three pizzas. Queen Margherita liked the pizza mozzarella the most, which is a pizza topped with red tomato sauce, white mozzarella, and green basil leaves (the same colors as the Italian flag). This pizza has been called pizza Margherita ever since. The pizza that she hated we now call Little Caesars.

Pizza continued to evolve over time. As Italians immigrated to the United States, they brought their pizza making skills with them. The first pizzeria in the United States sprung up on Spring Street in New Work City. Lombardi's opened in 1905 with a coal fired oven.

While New York may have the best pizza in the country, pizza spread to other large cities in America as well. Cities with large immigrant populations from Naples, like New York, Boston, Chicago, and Sing Sing Prison. However, pizza didn't become popular until after World War 2 as the troops came back from Europe with a newly found taste for pizza.

Beginning in the 1940's, pizza spread throughout United States. In 1943, Pizzeria Uno was started in Chicago. In 1958, Pizza Hut started in Wichita, Kansas. In 1967, Domino's opened its first restaurant. In 1984, Papa John's opened for business.

Pizza is now the most popular food in the country. But is pizza just junk food, or is there any nutritional value to pizza?

NUTRITIONAL BENEFITS OF PIZZA

Ever since the low-fat craze that swept the nation, pizza has been labelled as bad for you. In Italy however, pizza is considered an artisanal product. In America it's called junk food.

Pizza isn't junk from a nutritional standpoint. Pizza is good for you and is a great source of nutrients. Pizza can be a well-balanced meal and can easily contain foods from all four food groups.

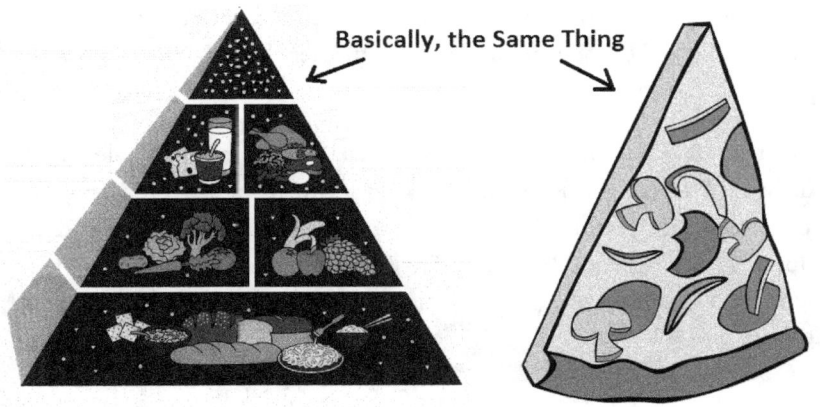

Basically, the Same Thing

Let's take a look at each component of pizza and their health benefits.

The basic building block of pizza is the dough. Pizza dough in its purest form is just flour, water, salt, and yeast. Pizza dough uses flour with more protein than all-purpose flour or bread flour. Pizza dough has vitamins A, B6, E, K, thiamine, riboflavin, niacin, pantothenic acid, folate, folic acid, lutein and zeaxanthin. Pizza dough also contains antioxidants from the chemical reactions of the yeast.

The next layer on pizza is the sauce. Tomato sauce contains 18 amino acids and the minerals it contains include calcium, iron, magnesium, phosphorus, potassium, sodium, zinc, copper, manganese and selenium. Tomato sauce also contains vitamins A, C, E, K, thiamine, riboflavin, niacin, pantothenic acid, vitamin B6, folate, choline, and lutein. But let's skip over all those and focus on one vitamin in particular: lycopene. This is where the real pizza nutritional magic happens.

Tomato sauce is rich in lycopene, a powerful antioxidant which helps fight against heart disease and many types of cancer. You read that correctly. Pizza can help fight against heart disease and cancer! Studies have found that eating pizza at least once a week may reduce the chances of getting stomach, colon, mouth, prostate, esophageal, and lung cancer.

Pizza is a great source of lycopene as tomatoes processed into sauce have more lycopene. Tomato sauce that is heated and combined with a small amount of fat, like mozzarella cheese, further boosts the amount of lycopene you absorb.

The next layer on pizza is cheese. Mozzarella cheese has a whole slew of vitamins: A, B12, D, E, K, thiamine, riboflavin, niacin, pantothenic acid, folate, choline and retinol. Cheese, of course, is also a great source of calcium. Calcium reduces the possibility of colon cancer. Mozzarella cheese contains iron, magnesium, phosphorus, potassium, sodium, zinc, copper, manganese and selenium.

The final layer of pizza is toppings. These have all kinds of nutritional value. Meat toppings like pepperoni, sausage, and beef are good sources of protein. Onions are rich in vitamin C, chromium, fiber, and help lower blood sugar and cholesterol. Black olives help fight heart disease, and lower cholesterol. Red peppers are a source of vitamins A, C, and B6. Olive oil reduces bad cholesterol and increase good one and prevent heart diseases. Garlic is rich with selenium, manganese, vitamin C and other beneficial compounds. Oregano is a good source of vitamin K, manganese, fiber and oils. I could go on and on listing all of the topping and health benefits, but I think you get the idea.

If you add all of this up, you get a yummy meal that contains numerous vitamins and minerals. Plus, pizza makes you happy. And as an added bonus pizza also fights heart disease and cancer.

Let's top this chapter off with a few pizza jokes.

TOP 10 PIZZA JOKES:

1. What's the difference between a pizza and my jokes? My pizza jokes can't be topped.
2. What's the difference between the pizza guy and the pizza? The pizza can feed a family of four.
3. To gain weight, takeaway Pizza. To lose weight, take away Pizza.

4. Why did the man get into the pizza business? He needed some dough.
5. Why did the hipster burn his lip? He ate pizza before it was cool.
6. What do you call a pizza lover? A dough nut.
7. A pizza walked into a bar. The bartender said, "Sorry, we don't serve food."
8. A pizza was waiting in the stomach to be digested. Suddenly a whiskey comes along. Pizza lets it pass by. Two minutes later another whiskey comes though. Pizza lets it pass by too. Then a couple minutes later, another whiskey comes along. This time pizza asks "What's going on out there?" The whiskey replies "They're having a party!" "Really?" says pizza, "I think I'll go check it out!"
9. The one thing about pizza jokes… It's all in the delivery.
10. Want to hear more pizza jokes? Nah, they're too cheesy.

FAKE TESTIMONIAL #7
PETE ZARIA: **YOU ARE WHAT YOU EAT- THAT'S WHY I SWITCHED TO THIN CRUST**

My diet consists mostly of salad. It's a simple salad with a big crouton, a lot of tomatoes, and topped with cheese. Ok… it's pizza. I don't eat salad, but I love pizza! Unfortunately, pizza doesn't love me. Although I'm not fat, I kind of look like a pizza. A large round pizza.

I knew I needed to lose weight. I weighed 300 pounds and I would get out of breath just talking on the phone ordering a pizza for delivery.

I've always believed the saying, "you are what you eat." I love pizza so much; I don't mind being a pizza. However, I didn't want to be a deep dish – I wanted to be a thin crust.

I knew if I was serious about losing weight, I should get professional help. I went to several nutritionists, but none of them would help me lose weight with a pizza diet. They all wanted me to eat a balanced diet with lots of fruit and vegetables. I told them that I don't mind a few fruit and vegetables as long as they're on top of a sauce covered crust and covered in melted mozzarella cheese. They just shook their heads in disgust. They told me I was out of shape. I told them that round is a shape.

I did the next best thing to actual medical and nutritional advice. I did an internet search. I discovered the Contrarian Diet. I really liked the emphasis on pizza as a diet food. I learned that pizza is a balanced meal, especially when you have a slice in each hand. Pizza can have all of the food groups: the crust is bread, the cheese is dairy, and the toppings can be meat, fruit, and veggies. What other food is so versatile?

I live in Chicago, so I eat a fair amount of deep dish pizza. By fair amount, I mean eating deep dish pizza on a daily basis. I knew I needed to make a change, otherwise I'd always look like a thick crust pizza. So I gave up thick crust and switched to thin crust.

I haven't actually lost any weight yet, but I do feel better about the pizza I eat. The Contrarian Diet helped me make a major change in my diet. I know it's just a matter of time before I thin out. In the meantime, I'll keep enjoying eating pizza.

Chapter 8

CANDY, IS IT DIABETES YET?

"Avoid any diet that discourages the use of hot fudge. "- Don Kardong

"I lied on my Weight Watchers list. I put down that I had 3 eggs... but they were Cadbury chocolate eggs." - Caroline Rhea

Trick or Treat?

Candy is both one of the most loved and most despised things we can eat. It's viewed as both a source of happiness and a guilty indulgence.

Candy is loved by every kid in the entire world, and maybe even in the entire Milky Way. At the same time candy has a long list of haters: dentists, physicians, school board members, Michelle Obama, and the mean lady down the street that hands out little boxers of raisins on Halloween.

So is candy a yummy treat to love and enjoy, or is it a teeth rotting, empty calorie, diabetes-causing evil that we should rid ourselves of once and for all?

I think candy is just misunderstood. You've been told all your life that candy is bad. But reality is that candy is good, unless of course you take it from strangers.

Why do you think candy is bad for you? Well, probably because you we told it's bad for you. There are so many misconceptions about candy. Let's unwrap the myths about candy and see if candy really is as bad as you believe.

MYTH #1: CANDY WILL ROT YOUR TEETH

Nope. Candy is no worse at causing cavities than many other foods. Cavities aren't caused by sugar, but rather by bacteria in your mouth. The bacteria feasts on the food left on your teeth. Eating fruit can lead to cavities as easily as eating candy. If you're worried about cavities, I think a good solution is to keep eating candy and start brushing your teeth.

MYTH #2: CANDY MAKES YOU FAT

Not true. Saying candy makes you fat is no different than saying broccoli makes you fat. Excess calories, not candy, makes you fat. You can get fat eating vegetables too, if you eat more calories than you need.

Plus, candy isn't even high in calories. A butterscotch candy only has 20 calories. 8 jelly beans have 115 calories. A cup of candy corn has fewer calories than a cup of raisins. Take that - mean lady down the street that doesn't give out candy to treat-or-treaters!

The National Confectioners Association, the experts on candy (and certainly not-bias when it comes to the nutritional value of candy), states that a study of more than 15,000 American adults found that people who ate candy did not have a higher weight or BMI.

A similar study at Louisiana State University (is that an Ivy league school?) tracked more than 11,000 American children aged 2- 18 from 1999 to 2004. Although tracking children sounds really creepy, the research showed that the children who ate candy were 22 percent less likely to be overweight than those who did not eat candy. For candy-eating adolescents, the rate was even higher, as they were 26 percent less likely to be overweight.

That kind of goes against everything you've been told. It looks like fat kids don't eat candy and the skinny kids do. Do you still think candy is bad for you?

MYTH #3: CANDY ISN'T REAL FOOD

Yes it is. Food is stuff you eat. People eat candy. Candy is food.

People have a hard time accepting candy as food because they have a difficult time placing candy into one of the four food groups. However, it's actually quite easy to place candy in one of the four food groups. Candy is a vegetable. Candy is mostly sugar, which is derived from either sugar cane or sugar beets – both of which are vegetables. Chocolate is also a vegetable. It's comes from sugar and cacao beans. Cacao beans come from a plant and are therefore vegetables. Nice time you hear, "eat your veggies," grab a chocolate bar.

MYTH #4: CANDY IS HIGH IN SUGAR

OK, this one is actually true, and not a myth. Aren't you a smartie. But are sugary foods really a problem?

If sugar is the problem, we have a lot of sugar in other food, like ketchup and jam. I don't hear people calling strawberry jam a junk food.

If you look at nutrition bars, they are essentially a candy bar with vitamins added. Health nuts have double standards. They go to the gym and buy nutrition bars, but then you hear snickers and get judgmental looks when someone is eating a candy bar. They're the same thing.

Also, candy isn't that different than the sugary fruit juice that many consider part of a healthy diet. Parents will give their kids a sippy cup of juice, but gasp if their kid is caught eating a piece of chocolate.

Some may argue that Americans eat too much sugar. That may be true, but candy isn't to blame. Candy only provides 6% of the added sugar in the American diet, while sweet drinks and juice supply 46%. If you really want to cut back on sugar, lay off the juice, not the candy.

MYTH #5: CANDY CAUSES DIABETES

That one is a real whopper! Even the American Diabetes Association states that eating too much candy causes diabetes is just a myth. Yet, you still hear people warn you that you'll go into a diabetic coma after eating a bag of candy.

MYTH #6: CANDY MAKES KIDS HYPERACTIVE

It doesn't. Researchers have shown that sugar doesn't cause hyperactivity. Kids often become hyper when they're having fun, like at birthday parties or on Halloween. While there is sugary food present at these events, a correlation isn't necessarily a cause. It could be that kids are just high off all the meds they take for ADHD, but it's definitely not the sugar that causing them to be hyper.

MYTH #7: CANDY IS JUST EMPTY CALORIES.

No. Other than hollow Easter bunnies, candy isn't empty calories. Keep reading and you'll discover the health benefits of candy.

HEALTH BENEFITS

Now that we know that candy isn't as bad as you think, is it actually healthful? Yes, candy does provide health benefits. There are mounds of evidence that candy is both nutritious and delicious.

A comprehensive study from the Harvard School of Public Health found that people who ate candy live longer than those that don't. The study revealed that people who ate a good and plenty amount of candy each month lived almost a year longer than those who ate no candy. The study credited phenol, the antioxidant which is also found in red wine, to be responsible for the increased longevity. It's your choice. If you want your kids to live longer, you can feed them candy or let them drink wine.

Candy can do more than just prolong your life. Here's a sampling of some candy and the health benefits they provide:

GUM

Studies show that chewing gum can reduce stress, improve mental health, and increase your alertness.

SKITTLES

A little known fact is that Skittles contain Vitamin C. Not only can you taste the rainbow, but you also can fend off scurvy, regulate blood sugar levels, get an antioxidant, and bolster your immune system by eating Skittles. Oh, and it also helps reduce the risk of cancer.

LICORICE

Licorice can help with memory problems associated with Type 2 diabetes, according to a 2011 study. Or was that a 2012 study? I can't remember, but either way, the study found that glabridin, a flavonoid in licorice, reversed learning and memory problems caused by Type 2 diabetes. Or was it Type 1 diabetes?

TOOTSIE ROLLS

Tootsie rolls apparently help with fatigue. An old advertisement for Tootsie Rolls claimed, "Eat Tootsie Rolls – The Luscious Candy that Helps Beat Fatigue." I don't know if it actually works, but if it was advertised it must be true. If you're in a crunch and need a little pick-me-up, try a Tootsie Roll.

COTTON CANDY

In addition to its superior properties as insulation in attics and walls, cotton candy can be used to restore and even create new blood vessels. Researchers at Cornell University claim that cotton candy can be melted down to create artificial blood vessels. Talk about having sugar running in your veins.

BLUE M&M'S

The blue food dye in blue M&Ms may be able to reduce spinal cord damage. Researchers at the University of Rochester Medical Center discovered that when they injected lab mice suffering from spinal cord injuries with the compound Brilliant Blue G (BBG), they were able to walk again. Although, the mice did walk with a limp, and temporarily turned blue. They also started humming an annoying song that went "La, La… La, La, La La…"

RAISINETS

According to Fitness magazine, chocolate-covered raisins, like Raisinets, can boost antioxidants and fiber. The movie industry also claims that eating Raisinets makes watching movies more enjoyable.

PEPPERMINT CANDY

Peppermint candy has so many health benefits that you'd think it would be considered medicine rather than food. Believe it or not, many universities have done studies on the benefits of peppermint. You'd think that universities would be studying the effects of beer, not peppermint. Maybe they eat peppermints to cover up their beer breath before they drive home. I'm not really sure why they'd study peppermint.

A Wheeling Jesuit University study states that peppermint candy makes drivers more alert. There's another reason to eat a peppermint on your way home from the bar. It not only covers up your beer breath, but it might save your life as you're more alert.

The Cornell Center for Materials Research states that peppermint oil contains higher levels of antioxidants than fruits and vegetables. Peppermint candy has antioxidant effects, as long as it's made with peppermint oil and not artificial flavors. If you're concerned about antioxidants and being healthy, but you hate fruits and veggies, then peppermint may be your solution.

A study at the University of Cincinnati suggests that peppermint can also help people concentrate better when taking tests. So can getting a good night's sleep. I guess if you didn't do that, just eat a peppermint during your test.

Peppermint candy can also help with digestion and stomach aches, as the peppermint oil can ease gas and bloating and an upset stomach. It may also help with heartburn and motion sickness.

Peppermint can cure bad breath, also known as halitosis. While other types of mints just cover up bad breath, peppermint actually cures it by destroying the bacteria that causes bad breath. It may also help prevent tooth decay and gum disease. You may want to give us brushing your teeth and just eat peppermints instead.

CHOCOLATE
If you were impressed by peppermint candy, wait until you see the health benefits that chocolate provides. Chocolate is the most healthful candy, bar none. It can be a lifesaver!

Chocolate can suppress coughing, act as an anti-depressant, boost good cholesterol in people with Type 2 diabetes, combat cancer, and protect your skin again harmful UV rays.

Chocolate, especially dark chocolate, can also decrease your risk of cardiovascular disease as chocolate is packed with powerful heart-healthy antioxidant flavonoids. Research shows that people that eat chocolate are 39% less likely to have a heart attack. Other research shows that chocolate eaters are 70% less likely to have a stroke, whether it's a swimming stoke, a tennis stroke, or a golf stroke. And even further research shows that chocolate eaters are 95% more likely to break out with acne.

ALL CANDY

Candy can restore willpower. The secret ingredient in candy that makes this happen is sugar. Kelly McGonigal, Ph.D., wrote in Psychology Today, "Studies show that when your blood sugar drops, your brain is less able to focus and control your impulses. But a small snack that increases blood sugar helps the brain snap back into self-control mode." If you don't have the willpower to avoid candy, try eating candy.

So in this chapter we established that candy isn't nearly as bad for you as you thought. In fact, candy has many surprising health benefits. To wrap up this chapter, consider not only the health benefits of candy but also the financial savings of a diet rich in candy. Candy is cheaper than Jenny Craig.

FAKE TESTIMONIAL #8
DENNIS TOFFICE: **I LEARNED HOW TO EAT A NUTRITIOUS, BALANCED MEAL**

Heart disease and stroke runs in my family. I had recently turned 50, so I wanted to take some major steps in preventing a heart attack or stroke.

I read the Contrarian Diet and learned that dark chocolate prevented cardiovascular disease, so started eating a chocolate bar after every meal. After breakfast, I ate a candy bar. Dark chocolate, of course. After lunch, I ate another candy bar. After dinner, I had a third candy bar. I did this every single day, but purely for medicinal purposes.

The side effect of this tasty medication is that I gained a few pounds (I also lost a couple teeth). They don't disclose that on the candy bar wrapper, but supposedly eating several chocolate bars a day can cause you to gain weight. I went to my doctor to find out what I was doing wrong.

Doc said that I shouldn't be eating so many chocolate bars. He said that I need to eat a balanced diet. It sounded too complicated to me. But, he taught me that eating a nutritious meal can be simple. Just look at your plate. You want to see lots of colors.

That sounded easy enough. I went home and filled my plate with lots of colors, just like the Doc ordered. I had red, yellow, green, and some other colors. I had filled my plate with M&Ms and Skittles.

I could still get all the health benefits of eating chocolate, plus I had a variety of colors on my plate. This was perfect. In my opinion, candy is the perfect food. A lot of candy is fat-free, it requires no refrigeration, it's relatively low in calories, it's inexpensive, and it tastes really, really good!

One of the surprising things about candy is the low calorie content. A side of Caesar salad can have 175 to 250 calories. People are fine with eating salad. No one says, "Hey, you need to cut back on salad. That's making you fat!" But they do say that about candy. But a Snickers bar has only 215 calories. A Hershey's milk chocolate bar has only 210 calories. That's actually less than many salads. Eating candy is actually a better diet than eating salad.

I'm still waiting to see my weight drop. However, I just feel so much better knowing I'm eating nutritious and balanced meals. I don't worry about heart attacks and strokes as much now that I'm eating right. I just love the Contrarian Diet. Thank you Contrarian Diet!

Chapter 9

LISTEN TO YOUR BODY

"I believe every human has a finite number of heartbeats. I don't intend to waste any of mine" – *Neil Armstrong*

"Aerobics: a series of strenuous exercises which help convert fats, sugars, and starches into aches, pains, and cramps." – *Unknown*

LISTEN TO YOUR BODY

Have you ever stopped to simply listen to your body? Yes, it sounds like a ticking time bomb. That's just your heart beat.

Our bodies are amazing. They let us know when things are good, like when we're reading a funny book we get happy and laugh. Our bodies also let us know when something is bad. If we step in hot lava, we feel pain and quickly move our foot (or what's left of our foot).

We have feelings, instinct, reflexes, and a conscious for a reason. Our bodies protect us. They give us warnings when we try to do something stupid or dangerous. When we ignore these warnings, bad things happen.

For example, when we get too close to the edge of a cliff, we get nervous and get back away. If we ignored this natural response, we could find ourselves plummeting to our death.

Why is it, when it comes to dieting, we think ignoring our body is a good idea? We put things in our mouth, like green veggie smoothies, that make us want to either gag or throw up. We exercise with the motto "no pain, no gain." We blatantly ignore all the warning signs that our bodies are sending to us.

Our body tells us to stop. But we insist on jogging five miles. Our mouth says, "I want ice cream," but we feed it salad. Is ignoring the messages from our bodies a good idea, or are we asking for trouble? Why do nutritionists and "diet experts" keep pushing the ideas that fly in the face of what our bodies tell us not to do?

IF IT HURTS, STOP.

"No pain, no gain" is simply bad advice. When your body hurts it's telling you something is wrong. If you ignore the pain you can do serious damage to your body.

If you're taking a walk around the block, and by the time you get to the end of your driveway your knee hurts, it's good to stop, turn around, and go back inside your home.

If you're walking up a flight of stairs and you get dizziness, nausea, or shortness of breath, it's time to take the elevator because you're probably going into cardiac arrest.

If you get out of breath bending over to tie your shoes, you should probably stop. If you get winded just saying the word "exercise," then quit talking. You're probably pushing yourself too hard. Sit down on the couch, eat a bag of chips, and watch soap opera re-runs. You don't want to strain your body and hurt yourself.

Pushing your body beyond its limits is a bad idea. Your body sends you pain as a way of saying "STOP!"

You should listen.

IF YOU'RE HUNGRY, EAT

Don't starve yourself to lose weight. If you quit eating, the first thing to go is your muscle. While you may weigh less, you're still fat. You just lost your muscle. The goal isn't to lose weight, but rather to lose fat. Ignore the bathroom scale and make sure to eat.

Food is fuel. Your body needs food just like a car needs gasoline. Don't let your body run out of fuel. Keep your energy up by eating when your body tells you it's hungry. If you choose not to eat, you'll slowly get hungry (and fast).

There is no reason to count calories or points. Even the president of Weight Watchers admitted that counting calories doesn't work. If you

68

resort to calorie counting, 250 calories of celery sticks is equivalent to 250 calories of a candy bar. Obviously these don't have the same health benefit. The candy bar is clearly the better choice.

IF YOU FEEL TIRED, SLOW DOWN

One of the common misconceptions about weight loss is that you should be active and exercise regularly.

Exercise uses energy. When your body is getting low on energy it gets tired. It's a bad idea to keep pushing yourself when you get tired. It's like trying to drive a car that is almost out of gas.

The problem with getting tired is that your body needs energy to break down fat and lose weight. If you push yourself too much by being active, you'll essentially turn off the weight loss switch. If you want to lose weight, you need to relax and preserve your energy for losing weight, not run marathons.

IF IT TASTES GOOD, EAT IT.

Other diets say "if it tastes good, it must be bad for you." Wrong!

Animals have the ability to sense nutrients in food. You don't see an ape reading nutrition labels. It just peels the banana and eats it. Deer don't worry about their blood pressure. They seek out salt licks and enjoy the sodium. Their body tells them they have a sodium deficiency and they hunger for it. People, like animals, also have the natural ability to detect nutritious food.

Your body knows the nutrition it needs and will literally hunger for it. It also knows what things are bad for it. The body's natural way of telling us it needs the nutrition from a particular food is to let us know that it tastes good. If you put honey in your mouth, you're body says "yum!" You should eat it.

Likewise, your body has a natural defense mechanism for warding off bad food. If you put some tree bark in your mouth, your body says "yuck!" You shouldn't eat it.

Think about things you shouldn't eat for a moment, like tree bark, grass, ear wax, or mud. They taste horrible. And they taste horrible for a reason. Your body is telling you that those things are dangerous to eat.

Now think about things that taste good, like honey, cheeseburgers, pizza, cake, pies, cookies, ice cream, and nachos. These taste good for a reason too. Your body craves them because it needs the nutrition.

Everyone's body is different and has different needs. Our warning system is the same – taste. Our tastes may be different, but if your body is telling you "yuck!" be careful and don't eat that food. This is where all other diets fail miserably. They try to unnaturally force you to eat things that your body doesn't want. If salad, celery, broccoli, and such taste bad to you, then avoid them.

Taste consolidates a complex assortment of dangers and simplifies it into one measurement. There is no need to read nutritional labels or lists of what to eat and what to avoid. Your tongue will let you know what nature intends for you to eat. It's simple: If it tastes good, eat it. If it tastes bad, spit it out.

IF IT FLIES, IT DIES!
Oops, that advice came out of the Bird Hunter's Manual. Sorry about that. Wrong book.

EAT FAST
You've heard that you should eat slowly because it takes time for your body to realize that it's full. So, if you eat slowly, you'll end up eating less.

That's just bad logic. Eating slow will allow you to eat significantly more over time than in a 10 minute sitting. The average American eats 1,996 pounds of food every year. That's nearly a ton of food. If you piled up a ton of food and gave the World champion hot dog eater 10 minutes to quickly eat as much as he can, he'd barely make a dent in the pile of food.

On the other hand, you could take a slow eater and let them look at it, poke at it, slowly put it in their mouth and savor every bite, and they could easily eat nearly a ton of food over the course of the next year. You can clearly eat more if you eat slowly.

Secondly, the idea that it take 20 minutes for your body to realize it's full implies we have defective bodies. If I poke you in the eye, does it take a while for your body to recognize pain? No, you feel it instantly. If you step into an outhouse, does it take your body 20 minutes to realize that it smells like a dairy farm? No, you immediately plug your nose. If you put a lemon in your mouth, is there any sort of a delay in your body realizing that you are tasting something sour? Of course not! Our bodies give us immediate feedback.

Your body knows when it's hungry, and it knows when it's full. Why would our bodies provide us immediate feedback on everything else, like when something hurts, we need to use the restroom, or something smells bad, but have a delayed reaction in letting us know when we're full. It doesn't make sense.

The other thing that doesn't make sense is thinking a person who eats for 30 minutes ends up eating less than a person who eats for only 5 minutes. The only way eating slowly will cause you to eat less is if you have a big family. I say eat fast and scarf your food down in 5 minutes. You'll get full faster and end up eating less. The guy that sits at the table slowly eating will eat a whole lot more.

It's kind of like boiling a frog. If you slowly turn the heat up, you can boil a frog. If you turn the heat up quickly, the frog will jump out. Eating slowly will cause you to eat more, not less. I don't really know how the frog analogy applies, but it sounds good.

WHY EXERCISE IS BAD

Everything you read or hear about exercise seems to be good. Everyone raves about how good exercise is for you. Yet we never hear the downside of exercise.

Everything has a downside, doesn't it? Sure living next to a nuclear plant is great because you get cheap electric bills and it creates jobs, but there's also a downside.

This chapter will explore the downside of exercising. It will show you, as a Contrarian dieter, why you should avoid exercise. Most people don't need excuses not to exercise. But just in case you're an exercise nut, here are three good reasons to avoid exercise:

1. Listen to your body – it doesn't like exercise.
2. Exercise is wasted energy.
3. Exercise is dangerous.

We've already discussed the idea of listening to our bodies. I don't know about your body, but my body doesn't like exercise. It doesn't like walking upstairs and it certainly doesn't like the idea of running marathons.

EXERCISE IS WASTED ENERGY

Americans are notoriously wasteful. We hear about how we waste food, waste money, and waste time. But we don't hear about one of the most wasteful activities we do – exercise.

In the past, people didn't need to exercise. They were active during the day. If you worked, you probably toiled in the farm, or worked hard with your hands making something. If you shopped, you probably walked around town. When kids played, they went outside and ran, jumped, and did other physical activities.

Thanks to the automobile, the TV, and the internet, people aren't nearly as active anymore. We drive just about everywhere we go rather than walk. We sit in cubicles or offices in front of a monitor at work. We stay home sitting on the couch watching TV. We don't go to the bookstore anymore to purchase books. We just download them off the internet like lazy people.

Many people decide that since they aren't as active anymore, that they should exercise. Exercise, however, is spending energy for the sole purpose of burning calories. It doesn't accomplish anything productive.

You may say that exercise is productive in that it improves your health and may contribute to weight loss. However, these are the possible effects of exercise, not something productive. If you walk from your house to the store, that's productive. Your physical activity provided a means of transporting you from one location to the next. If you walk on the treadmill, you produced nothing for the energy you spent. If you help a friend move by lifting heavy boxes, you are productive. If you lift weights in a gym, you are just wasting energy. It's funny how you can't find anyone to help you move, but you can find people that want to go to the gym with you and lift weights.

Exercising at a gym is like filling your car full of gas and driving around in circles. It's pointless and wasteful.

There is only so much energy. The sun provides energy to allow food to grow. We eat the food to keep our bodies alive. This food contains calories that allow us to do things, like walk, run, jump, lift heavy things like pianos. The amount of energy is limited. Yet, we treat energy as if it was an unlimited resource.

What would the world be like if people used the energy they wasted at the gym on productive things, like picking up litter, helping a friend move, or writing off-the-wall diet books. That wasted energy could actually be used for something productive.

EXERCISING IS DANGEROUS

Like much of our understanding of diet and nutrition, we accept many things about exercise based on what we've been told. Almost everyone thinks that exercise is good for you. The so-called experts tout exercising as healthful and claim that you will live a happier and longer life if you exercise regularly. Millions of Americans accept this advice on blind faith. After all, exercising isn't fun, so it must be good for us.

But where's the evidence that exercising actually leads to a happier, longer life? What if the experts are wrong? Why don't we hear about the dangers of exercising?

The experts have a reason to back exercising. Fitness is a multi-billion dollar a year industry. Of course you're going to be told that exercise is good for you. People want you to sign up for gym memberships, buy exercise equipment, buy workout clothing and shoes, subscribe to their health magazines, and buy their useless diet books like this one. There is a strong bias for people to tell you that exercise is good for you, because it's profitable for them.

Granted, there may be some benefits to exercising in moderation, however no one talks about the dark side of exercising. The simple truth is that exercising can lead to serious injury, illness, and even death. Let's take a look at the hidden risks of exercising.

EXERCISE WON'T MAKE YOU SKINNY

Many people have body perception disorders and use exercise, not to gain health, but rather to change their physical appearance to conform to society's expectations. They want to become skinny and believe that working out will shrink their body.

Vanity and exercising often go hand in hand. People can use exercise in order to fix parts of their body that they don't find acceptable. They become excessively concerned about their muscles being too small, their waist not being thin enough, or their spare tire looks like it would fit on a semi-truck. They exercise to the extreme in order to sculpt their body into the way they think it should look. They don't have a healthy view of their body and have never learned to accept their body the way it is.

Other people use exercise as a way to try to lose weight. This usually backfires, as exercising can kill your diet. Yes, exercising burns calories which in theory could cause you to lose weight, however exercising also increases your appetite. You eat more when you exercise. That doesn't help your diet. The more you exercise, the more you'll want to eat. Exercising isn't the way to get skinny and drop pounds. In fact, exercising will probably build your muscle which will add weight.

ADDICTIVE

Just like caffeine, cigarettes, alcohol, meth, and reading, exercising can be highly addictive. Over exercising isn't just a time consuming hobby, rather it's more of a drug addiction. Regular, strenuous exercise produces endorphins, hormones that make you feel good. Endorphins are chemically similar to morphine. That's why many people work out so much. They're literally addicted to the "high" of working out.

Like any addiction, exercise can interfere with other areas of your life, or even take over your life. People who exercise excessively may be missing out on time with friends and family. Exercise taken to the extreme can end friendships, lead to divorce, and ruin your career.

INJURY

One of the selling points to exercising is that you'll live a healthier life. Yet, there are a lot of athletes walking around with knee braces, casts, and other injuries.

Imagine you woke up today and had two choices: the first is to exercise, and the second is to lounge around the house watching TV and eating ice cream. What choice is more dangerous? Exercising or not exercising? Exercising is much more dangerous than not exercising. The risks of being lazy and eating ice cream is possible brain freeze if you eat your ice cream too fast. But exercising can subject your body to all kinds of harm.

The major problem with exercising is that it needlessly risks injury. Whether you're an occasional visitor to the gym or a professional athlete, exercising can lead to serious injury. When you make your body walk, jog, run, jump, skip, hop, duck, dive, swim, slide, climb, roll, waddle, stagger, or swivel to and fro, you subject your body to the risk of a tremendous amount of physical harm. And what makes it worse is that people tend to exercise to extremes. They push themselves further and further, and this involves more and more risk of injury. Exercising to the point of injury isn't healthy. But even leisurely exercising, like a walk around the block, can lead to injury. You could easily twist your ankle, fall and break a bone, or even trigger a heart attack.

Every year thousands of people are injured by exercising. Exercising can cause injury and lead to surgery and hospitalization. People who exercise frequently sprain or twist their ankles, get shin splints, break bones, pull muscles, get bruises and cuts, and suffer heat exhaustion and dehydration. Just take a trip to the local Emergency Room or Urgent Care. If you need more proof, drive to the gym. Why do you think there are so many disabled parking spots in front of the gym?

Exercise can lead to more than just temporary injuries; it can also cause permanent injury, poor health, or even death. Frequent, strenuous exercise can lead to long term health issues that can harm the body, skeletal, cardiovascular, respiratory, immune, and hormonal systems.

INFECTIONS

Another blow to the argument that exercise is good for you is the risk of infection. Gyms and health clubs are dirty, sweaty, smelly places. We all know that you can get sick going to the hospital. The same applies to gyms. They're full of germs, bacteria, fungus, and viruses. The wet areas like the showers, bathrooms, swimming pools, and used towels are all breeding grounds for bacteria. So are the cardio machines, weights, workout mats, and benches that are covered in sweat. You can get anything from athlete's foot to E. coli to genital warts from a dirty gym.

SICKNESS

There is evidence that too much exercise can reduce immunity and may even make you sick. Generally, we think exercise is good for immunity. While a little exercise can boost immunity, too much exercise can actually lower immunity.

Exercise temporarily suppresses your immune system. Researchers have conducted experiments with mice that show the mice that had strenuous exercise where more likely to get the flu than mice than sat in front of a TV all day sipping beer and eating nachos.

One study found that 90 minutes or more of strenuous exercise lowers your immunity for up to 72 hours after exercising. It is thought that the immune system is weakened during exercise through the increase in white blood cells and stress-related hormones. If you exercise strenuously, you can get sick easier. This is true whether you're a gym rat or a laboratory rat.

ALLERGIES

Asthma affects 20 million Americans and results in about 5,000 deaths annually. While there are different causes and forms of asthma, one of them is exercise-induced asthma (exercise-induced bronchoconstriction) that is an inflammation of your airways that makes it difficult to breath triggered by strenuous exercise.

While many people jokingly claim to be allergic to exercise, for some people they really are allergic to exercise. Exercise can trigger anaphylaxis where

76

you could get hives, have trouble breathing, experience a drop in blood pressure, get dizzy, and pass out or even die.

LOSS OF MINERALS

When you exercise, you lose a lot of minerals through sweating and urinating. Some of these minerals are needed for things like keeping cartilage intact and healthy. I, for one, would like to keep my cartilage intact, so I try not to exercise, sweat, or urinate.

TRAUMA

Our bodies are able to move quickly as a result of nature. We have a natural "fight or flight" instinct. If we face danger, the flight instinct gives us the ability to move quickly. However, flight is designed to only be used rarely and only temporarily, not 30 – 60 minutes every day.

During "flight," our heart beat increases rapidly to deliver more needed oxygen, we breathe faster so that our lungs take in more oxygen, blood vessels are constricted as blood is fed to the brain and muscles, and adrenaline is pumped into the bloodstream.

If we only use the flight instinct occasionally, as it is designed, it helps us quickly escape danger. If we run or exert ourselves on a daily basis, we are forcing trauma on our bodies. Some studies suggest that strenuous exercise can lead to bad stuff.

Strenuous exercise increases oxygen utilization, which increases production of free radicals. This in turn causes oxidative damage to muscles and other tissues. Excessive exercise can cause significant free radical damage and leads to chronic systemic inflammation. Chronic inflammation is associated with cancer, heart disease, strokes, MS, Alzheimer's, Parkinson's, and premature aging. People usually exercise to avoid these things, not create these health issues.

DEATH

Exercising can even lead to death. There have been numerous reports of athletes that have collapsed and died. One of the risks of exercising is that is can trigger sudden cardiac death. Basketball players, football players, and marathon runners have all collapsed and died from heart attack or stroke while exercising. Jim Fix, author of The Complete Book of Running, who promoted running to prevent heart disease ironically collapsed and died while jogging from a heart attack.

Injuries from exercising are no laughing matter. We hear about weight lifters that literally pull their arms out of their sockets trying to lift too much weight. Every year we read about someone who was leisurely walking on their treadmill only to have the speed increase and shoot them back through a wall like a speeding bullet. We've seen reports on the evening news about joggers being ripped apart by blood thirsty packs of rabid raccoons. And we've all known victims of yoga that have left people permanently tied up in a pretzel-like condition unable to ever stand up straight again.

The idea that exercise can do more harm than good is surprising. But the fact is that exercising is extremely dangerous and it has left a trail of victims. Just don't be one of them. While society may frown on laziness, play it safe and throw in the gym towel.

FAKE TESTIMONIAL #9
JIM SARBAD: **I STOPPED EXERCIZING AND HAVEN'T BEEN TO THE E.R. EVER SINCE.**

I used to be an exercise nut. I would swim, bike, and run. I would work out every day for hours. I guess you would call me a gym rat. I always thought the gym was a good place for me, especially since my name is Jim. I would get to the gym before work and run on the treadmill. During lunch, I'd come back and lift weights. After work, I'd go to a yoga class or spin class. On the weekends, I'd spend time outside exercising. I use to work out all the time.

The problem is I used to get hurt a lot too. I've been beaten up after trash talking some guys at the community basketball court. I broke my ankle once when I was watching birds through my binoculars while jogging. That didn't stop me though. I didn't give up jogging until one day my thighs kept rubbing together and caught my pants on fire. I also nearly drown went I came up with the bright idea of tying weights to my arms and legs while swimming in order to build more strength. I also cracked my skull open

78

when I was lifting weights and working on my balance by standing on an exercise ball as I lifted.

I probably spent as much time in the hospital as the gym. The staff in the Emergency Room at my local hospital knew me by name. I'd come in injured, with like a sliver in my finger, a spangled ankle, or my family jewels on fire, and they'd ask me, "Jim, what did you do this time?"

Let's see, over the years I've broken both legs, had shin splints, separated my shoulder (twice), tore my ACL, sprained my wrist, jammed my finger (don't ask where), ruptured my Achilles tendon, fractured my ankle, had a torn router cuff (that hurt), pulled my hamstring, had a severe concussion (I think), fractured vertebrae, and had a lawn dart impaled in my skull (it's a long story, but it happened at the gym).

I knew I needed a major change in my life or exercise was going to be the death of me. One day in the E.R. waiting room, I saw a woman reading a book titled the Contrarian Diet. I was curious and also bored because I had looked at all of the hospital magazines already. I asked her about it and she said that the book recommended not exercising as a way to stay healthy.

I had always assumed that I needed to exercise to stay healthy. I never thought not exercising was good for you. Then I thought about all my trips to the E.R. Maybe this Contrarian Diet was on to something.

I bought my own copy of the Contrarian Diet and read it to the best of my limited reading ability. Basically, I read the cover, looked at the pictures, and then just remembered what the smart lady at the E.R. told me about the book. So, I stopped exercising.

I haven't been to the E.R. ever since. I feel so much healthier now that I don't work out in the gym. I joke about being in the Fitness Protection Program. I know society frowns on laziness, so I just quit calling my toilet John. I now refer to it as Jim. That way, every morning I can tell people, "I went to the Jim this morning."

I admit, sometimes I miss the gym, but then I just watch workout videos at home. I don't exercise as I watch them. I just sit on the couch eating ice cream cheering them on. It gives me the sense of working out, but I get to sit in the comfort of my own couch. I guess it's kind of like watching football. You can get into it, but there's no danger of getting tackled or hurt. You get to watch guys exercise and play ball while you drink beer and eat nachos. I do get off the couch now and then and go to the Jim. The Contrarian Diet has given me a whole new life – and it's a whole lot safer.

Chapter 10

BACK TO GASTROENTEROLOGY

"It is universally well known, That in digesting our common Food, there is created or produced in the Bowels of human Creatures, a great Quantity of Wind. That the permitting this Air to escape and mix with the Atmosphere, is usually offensive to the Company, from the fetid Smell that accompanies it." – Benjamin Franklin

"Beans, beans, the musical fruit: The more you eat, the more you toot! The more you toot, the better you feel: So let's have beans at every meal!" – School Children

As I mentioned, I developed the Contrarian Diet based on my work as a gastroenterologist. In an effort to develop a diet that would prevent my patients from excess flatulence, I became an expert on the risks of eating vegetables.

One of the big problems with other diets is that they push vegetables. Veggies can make you bloated, cause stomach pain, and make you rip some really big smelly farts. Let's take a look at the case against eating vegetables.

THE CASE AGAINST EATING RABBIT FOOD

If eating traditional sugary, salty, and fatty foods doesn't kill you, why do we eat salad and broccoli? Good question.

The Contrarian Diet discourages the consumption of vegetables. While veggies aren't forbidden, they are discouraged and often ridiculed. If you really want lettuce and tomato on your cheeseburger, that's your business. But, here is why the Contrarian Diet doesn't promote veggies.

First of all, avoiding veggies is a natural part of the Contrarian Diet because… well, it's contrarian. The main reason why the Contrarian Diet is anti-vegetable is because every other diet encourages eating veggies. It wouldn't be the Contrarian Diet is it wasn't contrarian.

The second reason, and perhaps the best, is that veggies taste bad. You shouldn't put anything in your mouth that tastes bad. Personally, I avoid putting the following in my mouth: food that fell on the floor, money (especially dollar bills), my fingernails, loaded guns, and of course... veggies.

The third reason not to eat veggies is that they make you fat. Why do you think they feed corn and grain to fatten up pigs and cows?

If the first three reasons weren't enough to convince you to avoid veggies, let's look at the health risks of eating vegetables. Yes, that's right - the health risks. No one talks about the health risk of vegetables, but surprisingly veggies may not be as good for you as you think.

Veggies can kill you. Ask any survivalist you know. He'd be the guy with all the canned food, guns, and bars of gold. What's safer to eat in nature, animals or plants? If they know anything about survival, they'll tell you that animals are safer to eat. Plants, in general, are poisonous. Between 90% to 95% of plants are poisonous. Meat, on the other hand, is generally safe to eat. Eating plants (a.k.a. veggies) not only is disgusting, but it can actually kill you.

Veggies also cause food poisoning. Every year 1 in 9 people in the U.S. gets food poisoning. That's 9 million people puking out their guts and sitting on the toilet with explosive diarrhea! What's the leading cause of food poisoning? You guessed it! It's raw leafy greens like spinach and lettuce. Mmm... tasty bacteria. Leafy greens can also cause E.Coli, salmonella, and listeria. Fruit and vegetables cause 46% of all food poisoning. That's about 4.5 million people in the U.S. getting food poisoning every year because they're eating their fruits and veggies. If the veggies don't kill you right away, you may wish you were dead after you get food poisoning.

Most of the benefits of eating veggies are bogus. You probably think eating carrots is good for your vision. Not according to an Ohio State University study that showed that some beta-carotene molecules block the body's absorption of vitamin A, which is essential for eye, bone, and skin health, as well as normal metabolism and immune function.

Talking about carrots, if you eat too many of them they can literally change the color of your skin orange. So can pumpkins.

Veggies can do strange things to your pee too. Eating asparagus can make your pee smell funny. Eating beets can change your pee a red color.

Veggies can also mess with your body is similar ways. If you eat tomatoes, you get heartburn. If you've ever eaten a bowl of spaghetti or a pizza and gotten heartburn, it's the acidic tomatoes that are to blame. If you're going to get heartburn, you might as well eat pizza.

If you sat down and ate a bunch of carrots, raw spinach, asparagus, beets, and tomatoes, it may sound like a nutritious meal. However, when you strand up you may have orange skin, heart burn, explosive diarrhea, and stinky bright red pee. It might just be me, but it doesn't sound like veggies are really good for you.

Don't get me wrong. Not all vegetables are bad. Processed veggies like potato chips, French fries, ketchup, etc. are fine. So are things that either sound like veggies like candy corn, or things that contain some veggies like carrot cake and pumpkin pie.

There really is no reason to put your life or your health at risk by eating veggies. Veggies aren't necessary. Ask any carnivore. Our ancestors had no other choice but to eat fruit and vegetables. They discovered that if you didn't eat them, you'd get scurvy. They didn't understand vitamins and that it was Vitamin C, not the fruit and vegetables, which prevented scurvy. We have alternatives now. We can take a daily multi-vitamin or eat a bowl of cereal. We don't need veggies.

Any diet that makes you eat veggies is just cruel and unusual. Eating veggies is also a major health risk that could lead to your early demise.

FART ATTACKS

Passing gas is normal. We general toot about 20 times a day. However, when you start eating a lot of veggies those toots become sonic blasts of stink that nobody enjoys.

Besides the uncomfortableness of bloating and stomach pain, explosive diarrhea, and socially embarrassing moments of passing gas, a veggie rich diet comes with a very real health risk.

Diet is crucial in preventing excess flatulence. The danger of eating the foods other diets recommend, namely vegetables, is that it causes a plaque buildup in your lower intestines. As we eat food, we also swallow some air. The body's natural way of releasing this air is through flatulence. However, if you eat too many vegetables and the plaque buildup in your lower intestine breaks off and prevents the flatulence from escaping your body, you could die from a fart-attack.

I firmly believe that preventing most fart-attacks is doable. The key on cutting down on flatulence is through proper diet. Asparagus, broccoli, Brussels sprouts, cabbage, and onions are all high flatulence producing vegetables that should be avoided, or at the very least eaten in moderation.

If you ignore this, you'll someday have to take your chances with the miracle of modern day medicine – Beano or Gas-X. These medications are an admission of failure. You failed to eat a diet that would prevent flatulence. These pills are the last ditch effort to cure your flatulence and help prevent future fart-attacks.

I believe in a prevention approach. It's better to avoid vegetables and stop flatulence before it starts, then eating vegetables and risk a fart-attack.

I'm a busy gastroenterologist, so needless to say I'm running a little behind. I won't bore you with all the scientific explanation of exactly how flatulence causes fart attacks. Just trust me when I say that you should avoid veggies. Let's finish up this up section of the chapter - I'm pooped.

FAKE TESTIMONIAL #10
BILL LEEAKE: **I HAVE A NEW BELT & I DON'T FART ANYMORE!**

I've had bad gas all my life. It kind of runs in my family. I know everyone passes gas, but I pass gas constantly. It's so bad that I've actually had a hard time dating, keeping friends, keeping steady employment, and keeping my underwear white.

My parents were always very flatulent as well. I just thought it was hereditary. We had a favorite joke in my family growing up. Why do they only put 239 beans in a can of Boston baked beans? Because if they added one more, it would be too farty.

I was raised eating lots of fresh fruits and vegetables. My mom would never let me eat candy or sweet deserts. If I wanted a snack, I'd get broccoli. If I begged for ice cream because the other kids in the neighborhood got to eat ice cream, I'd get a celery stick. On special occasions, like my birthday, I'd get to blow out the candles on a big plate of green beans.

Growing up with bad gas was difficult. The other kids at school made fun of me and called me Billy Stinky Butt. No one wanted to be my friend. I can understand why. I really did stink.

I always thought that was just who I was. Billy Stinky Butt. I guess I never knew any better. When I became an adult I kept eating fruits and vegetables. I would eat a bowl of fruit for breakfast along with non-fat yogurt, a salad for lunch, and rice and beans for dinner. I lived alone in a modular home, so it did matter how often I passed gas. I did set off the carbon monoxide alarm on a regular basis. I guess it detected a natural gas leak.

One day I was out shopping for new underwear and I started farting uncontrollably. There were a lot of other shoppers in the store and they all covered their faces, coughed, and gave me dirty looks as they ran out of the store in disgust. I know if other people hurt us, like those shoppers hurt my feelings, we're supposed to turn the other cheek. Somehow this just doesn't seem to be appropriate in my situation.

I guess that was the thing that caused me to seek help. I confessed my farting to my doctor and he referred me to a gastroenterologist. I explained to the gastroenterologist my genetic predisposition. He just laughed. He told me to quit eating so many fruits and vegetables, and he handed me a copy of the Contrarian Diet. He told me that I had suffered from a fart attack and that if I didn't change the way I was eating, I would possibly die from a fart attack.

I certainly didn't want to die from a fart attack. I was only 33 years old. I read the Contrarian Diet, stopped eating fruits and vegetables, and started eating ice cream, pizza, and candy. I noticed a major change almost immediately in my health, weight and lack of flatulence. I was cured!

Sure, I did gain a little weight and had to buy a new belt. But, it was worth it because I didn't stink anymore. Best of all, I feel so much better not having to worry if I'm going to have a fart attack in public. I just wish I would have discovered the Contrarian Diet earlier in life.

Chapter 11

Why People Don't Fail on the Contrarian Diet

"Probably nothing in the world arouses more false hope than the first four hours of a diet." – Dan Bennett

"Many a person who goes on a diet finds out in short order that they are poor losers." – Unknown

We've all know that annoying person that just started their diet. They're all excited about the new rules and restrictions and feel that they need to inform everyone they come in contact with about what their diet allows and doesn't allow. They're also excited about all the weight they're going to magically lose. Not only have they committed to changing their eating habits to this bizarre set of rules and regulations, but they also expect you and everyone else they know or meet to be on their diet as well.

You can spot a new dieter easily as they're the one commenting on everything you're eating and lecturing you about what and how you should eat. It sounds like this, "I can't believe you're eating that piece of bread. It's even white bread! That's so bad for you. That's pure carbs. And you put butter on it too! That's so bad for you. I can't eat bread. I make my sandwiches between two pieces of lettuce and can only eat them on Tuesdays and every other Thursday."

The new dieter will lose some weight initially, however most of the weight loss is just water weight from crying. This quick drop in weight gets them even more excited as they see the "results" of their self-starvation and insane alliance to some set of wacky eating rules. Encouraged, they continue their tortuous diet.

After a while, every dieter has the natural desire to eat real food. They crave sugar, carbs, sodium, and fat. They want to eat a fulfilling meal, not just veggie snacks. So they cheat a bit. They eat a slice of bread or a cracker. Of course, they love it. So they cheat a little bit more. This time it's something more like a box of a dozen donuts or an entire sheet cake. Now eating those lettuce sandwiches is really difficult. They cheat a little more. Soon, they are cheating more than they are dieting.

They feel horrible for cheating on the diet. Within a short few weeks, they've gone from a faithful dieter to a cookie monster that will devour everything in the kitchen. They also gained weight and now weigh more than when they started the diet. They feel like they failed the diet.

Not to give up, they decide to start the diet over again. It worked once. They did lose a little weight at first. This time they won't cheat. But they do cheat. And faster than the first time. Frustrated, burned out, feeling like a loser, and fatter than ever, they quit. Diets suck. This is how the typical diet tragically ends.

What if dieting didn't have to be so bad? The key to success on a diet all comes down to dietary adherence. The reason why all other diets fail is because their food sucks. That's what makes the Contrarian Diet different.

On other diets people lose weight temporarily, but regain more than they lost. They would have been better off not being on the diet. All that yo yo dieting just isn't good for you, especially when you get the string stuck in your teeth. Plus, that walk the dog trick isn't even real exercise.

The Contrarian Diet is different. People don't tend to fail on the Contrarian Diet. Other diets don't work because they're not sustainable. The Contrarian Diet, on the other hand, is very easy to sustain. The success of the Contrarian Diet all comes down to dietary adherence. You'll stick to a diet if you like its taste. People like the taste of sugar, carbs, sodium, and fat.

The Contrarian Diet allows you to eat bowls of ice cream, slices of pizza, bacon cheeseburgers, chocolate, and candy. You can drink beer and soda. You can eat cookies, cake, pies, bread, muffins, and plates full of pasta.

Why would anyone want to give up a diet that tastes so good? If you want a diet you can stick with, and I'm not talking about for a few weeks or even months. If you want a diet you can stick with for years or even a lifetime (however short that may be), there is no diet that has better dietary adherence than the Contrarian Diet.

No one enjoys being on a diet. No one enjoys being around someone who is on a diet. But the Contrarian Diet is different. It's almost like you aren't even on a diet.

Let's get real. Any diet that doesn't let you splurge on sugar, carbs, salt, and fat is going to fail. The Contrarian Diet is the only diet that allows you to eat all of these things in abundance. That's why it works. And that's why you'll love it.

Plus, it's fun to see the reactions of your friends when you're out for dinner and they order chicken and you eat all the bread and then order a large plate of fettuccine alfredo and a tiramisu for desert, and then you tell them you're on a diet. Or, when the waiter asks if you'd like salad and you simply say, "no thanks, I'm trying to cut back on veggies."

FAKE TESTIMONIAL #11
CLARA SABELL: **I WENT ON THE CONTRARIAN DIET AND LOST 15 POUNDS!**

Confessions first. I'm British and I bought the Contrarian Diet book and probably overpaid. I spent 15 pounds buying the daffy book.

I went on the Contrarian Diet because my husband heard about it at work. He was concerned about my health – I was 32 years old and weighted about 120 kilos. So as a Valentine's Day gift he bought me a copy of the Contrarian Diet and an exercise bike. Obviously he didn't read the Contrarian Diet or he would know that an exercise bike is useless. It's also an insulting Valentine's Day gift!

My weakness, other than stupid men, was quantity. That's quantity of food, not men. I ate a lot of food, but not really a lot of sweets. I snacked all the time. Donuts at breakfast, biscuits during the afternoon, crisps before supper, ice cream after supper, and a nosh or two before going to Uncle

Ned. OK, maybe I did eat a lot of sweets. When I got up in the night, I'd raid the refrigerator.

For meals I'd eat a lot too. Breakfast I'd eat bacon, sausage, eggs, baked beans, mushrooms, and fried bread. For lunch I'd grab some fish and chips. For supper I'd eat a big plate of curry rice or pasta.

When I read the Contrarian Diet I was all excited to start. Then I realized, I was basically already on the Contrarian Diet. I went over the three main things that would make up the Contrarian Diet. I ate anything I wanted. Check. I ate like a pig. Check. I didn't exercise. Check.

I had been on other diets before. I once was on a diet for a whole week. All I lost was seven days of my life that I'll never get back. I was excited that I was already on the Contrarian Diet. It had been over a year since my last diet flop. This meant that I had been on the Contrarian Diet for over a year. I didn't care if I hadn't lost any weight; I was just excited that I managed to stay on a diet for that long.

I told my mates (both of em) about my diet success. I described how the Contrarian Diet worked and that I had been on it for over a year without quitting. To my amazement, they both concluded that they also have been on the Contrarian Diet most of their lives and didn't even know it. Now I had diet mates. We could go eat chippy together!

That got me wondering. How many people are on the Contrarian Diet and don't even realize it?

Chapter 12: How to Really Lose Weight

Eat more. Move less.

PART II:
MEAL PLANS
AND RECIPES

Meal Plan

Phase 1 is by far the strictest, cruelest, suckiest part of the Contrarian Diet. The recipes for Phase 1 are actual recipes used for the inmates in San Quentin State Prison. Basically, all you can eat for the first week of the diet is bread and water. While Phase 1 is a high carb diet, you won't enjoy this part of the diet. There really is no reason to put you through Phase 1 other than we feel the need to torture you the first week of the diet in the time honored tradition of fad dieting.

Just kidding. You don't need to do Phase 1; this is the Contrarian Diet. This is the diet for people that actually like food. You'll enjoy extremely large portion sizes, and get to indulge in delicious food like ice cream, pizza, and candy.

Other diets have multiple phases. They start out with food you really hate and then ease up a bit as the diet progresses. You go from Phase One, to Phase Two, to Phase Three, and then you get frustrated, hungry, and depressed and you end the diet. Three phases and you're out.

The Contrarian Diet is completely different. There are no phases. On the following pages you'll be given a sample meal plan for a typical week on the Contrarian Diet along with the recipes. You don't need to follow this plan or make the recipes. The meal plan and recipes are here as examples and entertainment.

This is important. Don't eat all of the junk food in your house the day before you start the diet. The Contrarian Diet is unlike any diet you've tried before. You're actually going to need that junk food to make these recipes.

Cooking from recipes is kind of like using an online dating service. They never look as good as the pictures. So I didn't include any pictures of the food.

DAY 1

BREAKFAST
Donut
Breakfast Sandwich
Irish Coffee

MORNING SNACK
Brownie Ice Cream Sandwich

LUNCH
Cream Cheese, Bacon, & Caramelized Onion Hot Dog
Cream of Tomato Gorgonzola Soup
Long Island Ice Tea

AFTERNOON SNACK
Pepperoni Pizza Bites

DINNER
Double Bacon, Double Cheese, Double Mayo, Double Burger
Loaded Pub Waffle Fries
Twinkie Milkshake

DESSERT
Chocolate Cheese Cake
Bowl of ice cream

BEDTIME SNACK
Chocolate Chip Cookies

Day 2

Breakfast
Ooey, Gooey Cinnamon Rolls
Mimosa

Morning Snack
Peanut Butter Balls

Lunch
Loaded Macho Nachos
Mudslide

Afternoon Snack
Homemade Potato Chips

Dinner
Lasagna
Bacon Feta Beans
Soda or Beer

Dessert
Molten Chocolate Cake

Bedtime Snack
Chocolate Popcorn

DAY 3

BREAKFAST
Country Scones with Devonshire Cream
Bloody Mary

MORNING SNACK
Fudge

LUNCH
Deep Fried Peanut Butter & Jelly Sandwich
Soda

AFTERNOON SNACK
Soft Pretzels

DINNER
Fettuccine Alfredo
Snickers Salad
Peanut Butter Cup Milkshake

DESSERT
Bananas Foster

BEDTIME SNACK
Church Stained Glass Windows

DAY 4

BREAKFAST
Home Made Chocolate Glazed Donuts
Soda

MORNING SNACK
More Home Made Chocolate Glazed Donuts
2 pints of Rocky Road ice cream

LUNCH
Garden Salad (just joking). Actually, Fluffernutter sandwich and a soda!

AFTERNOON SNACK
Pizza delivery . Order a large pepperoni and sausage pizza. If you're eating alone, yell "pizzas here" so that the pizza delivery guy doesn't think you're a loser.

DINNER
New York Style Pizza (you can never eat too much pizza)
Beer or soda

DESSERT
Brownie Sundae Topped with Maraschino Cherry

BEDTIME SNACK
Left over pizza

DAY 5

BREAKFAST
Mimosa
Irish Coffee

MORNING SNACK
Another round of Mimosa

LUNCH
Mocha Breve Breakfast Smoothie

AFTERNOON SNACK
Half a Bottle of Wine

DINNER
Big Ass Burrito
Long Island Ice Tea

DESSERT
Mudslide

BEDTIME SNACK
The Other Half of the Bottle of Wine

DAY 6?

LATE BREAKFAST
Cake Batter Pancakes & Ice Cream
A Couple Bloody Marys
Several Aspirin

LATE MORNING SNACK
Bacon, Egg, & Cheese Bagel

LUNCH
Bacon Butty
Soda

AFTERNOON SNACK
Chocolate Chip Cookies
Home Made Potato Chips

DINNER
Stromboli
3 Cheese & Bacon Macaroni & Cheese
Soda

DESSERT
Chocolate Sheet Cake

BEDTIME SNACK
Candy bar. Before you go to bed, make sure to set your scales back ten pounds. You'll need to do your weigh in tomorrow for the end of the first week of the Contrarian Diet.

DAY 7

BREAKFAST
Cinnamon Roll French Toast
Irish Coffee

MORNING SNACK
Fudge

LUNCH
Frosting Sandwich (really)
Long Island Ice Tea

AFTERNOON SNACK
Bowl of ice cream

DINNER
Sage Butter Gnocchi
Authentic Irish Mashed Potatoes
Soda

DESSERT
Mudslide

BEDTIME SNACK
Candy Bar and Soda

The Contrarian Diet Recipes

"The biggest seller is cookbooks and the second is diet books—how not to eat what you've just learned how to cook." — Andy Rooney

"A good cook never cooks carrots and peas in the same pot." - Unknown

Diet books have a little blurb at the beginning telling you how this new diet is going to allow you to lose a ton of weight, they tell you the do's and don'ts of the diet, and they mention their credentials (PhD, MD, etc.). Most of the book, however, is just a bunch of recipes, and crappy ones at that since they only let you eat certain foods.

Well, you've made it past the part of the book that tells you about this new miraculous diet. I've listed the do's and don'ts, so here is the part of the book that gives you the recipes that you can eat on this diet.

At least on the Contrarian Diet, the recipes taste really good.

Here are the best ooey gooey recipes chock full of sugar, salt, butter, bacon, and other artery-clogging ingredients.

If you mess up any of these recipes, don't worry. Just call and order a couple pizzas. They probably taste better than anything you can cook anyway, and are much more nutritious than most of the recipes in this book.

FOODS TO EAT

- Anything and everything. It is recommended, but not required, that you try to avoid the list of foods below.

FOODS TO AVOID
- Low-fat or non-fat cheese. Eat the real thing.
- Low-fat or non-fat milk or dairy products. Drink whole milk or cream.

- Human Placenta. For obvious reasons. Although people do eat this.
- Asparagus. It will make your pee smell funny.
- Beans, Broccoli, Brussels Sprouts, Cabbage, and Onions. These vegetables are known by the State of California to cause fart attacks. See Chapter 10.
- Celery. Don't fall for the trick where celery is topped with peanut butter and raisins and called "Ants on a Log". It's still celery and it's still disgusting.
- Mushrooms. Except psychedelic mushrooms.
- Spinach. Those Popeye cartoons were just propaganda to get kids to eat veggies.

Nutrition Facts

Serving Size 1 entire bag (1g)
Servings Per Container 1

Amount Per Serving

Calories 5100   Calories from Fat 4950

	% Daily Values*
Total Fat 188g	**289%**
Saturated Fat 94g	**470%**
Trans Fat 89g	
Cholesterol 897mg	**299%**
Sodium 6223mg	**259%**
Total Carbohydrate 512g	**171%**
Dietary Fiber 2g	**8%**
Sugars 200g	
Protein 1g	**2%**

*Percent Daily Values are based on a 2,000 calorie diet.

Warning: Nutritional information in the following recipes is not accurate and is sketchy at best.

SCONES WITH DEVONSHIRE CREAM

A tasty British treat. The Brits like to have a little fun with their left over scones as apparently scones are poisonous to birds. They leave them outside on their back porch. Sometimes they get lucky and kill two birds with one scone.

DEVONSHIRE CREAM:

8 ounces cream cheese, softened

½ cup sour cream (not the fat-free or low-fat crap)

2 tablespoons of fancy pants confectioners' sugar

SCONE:
2 cups all-purpose flour

1 tablespoon baking powder

1/4 teaspoon salt

4 tablespoon butter, diced

1 large egg (from a chicken, not an ostrich… it doesn't need to be that large)

5 tablespoons whole milk

1 large egg beaten to submission (to glaze the scones)

Make the Devonshire cream by whipping the cream cheese, sour cream, and confectioners' sugar until well mixed. Chill until serving.

Preheat the oven to 425 degrees F. Cover a baking sheet with butter.

Whisk the egg and milk together. Set aside.

In another bowl, whisk the flour, baking powder, and salt together and then cut in the butter. Add the cream mixture until it forms a soft dough.

Transfer the dough to a lightly floured surface and knead until the dough comes together. Roll out the dough to an inch thick, then cut into scone-shaped wedges.

Transfer to the baking sheet and brush the tops of the scones with the beaten egg.

Bake for 8 minutes or until golden.

Serves 3 (it only makes a dozen scones)

NUTRITION AT A GLANCE

Per serving: 1460 calories, 2 g protein,
181 g carbohydrates, 62 g fat, 36 g saturated fats,
1260 mg sodium, 215 mg cholesterol, 2 g fiber

CINNAMON ROLL FRENCH TOAST

This is an authentic French recipe from Paris. I like to pair this recipe with a glass of Romanée Conti and a few imported gourmet cheeses.

4 cinnamon rolls

½ stick melted butter (1/4 cup)

5 large eggs

½ cup heavy whipping cream

2 teaspoons ground cinnamon

2 teaspoons vanilla

1 cup chopped pecans

¾ cup maple syrup

Cut cinnamon rolls into bread size slices.

Preheat frying pan.

Whisk eggs. Using both hands and remembering to lift from your knees, pick up the heavy whipping cream and add it to the egg mixture. Then add the cinnamon and vanilla and whip.

Dunk cinnamon roll slices, one at a time, into the batter to cover them completely.

Add cinnamon roll slices to the frying pan. Cook in the frying pan until golden brown, about 2 minutes per side.

Remove French toast from frying pan and cover with maple syrup and pecans.

Serves 1

NUTRITION AT A GLANCE

Per serving: 1278 calories, 7 g protein,
169 g carbohydrates, 74 g fat, 52 g saturated fats,
1534 mg sodium, 316 mg cholesterol, 4 g fiber

DONUT BREAKFAST SANDWICH

For those that want to go beyond just eating donuts for breakfast, this sandwich takes breakfast to a whole new level. An early morning confectionery delight, you'll be sure to enjoy the contrast of the sugary donut with the salty egg. This breakfast sandwich will make your taste buds dance. It may also make you vomit if you eat it all, but don't worry about that.

　　1 glazed donut

　　Some butter

　　1 slice of your favorite cheese

　　2 slices of microwave bacon (the lazy person's way to fry up happiness)

　　1 large egg

　　1 tablespoon confectioner's sugar

　　Salt & pepper to taste

Microwave bacon per instructions on packaging.

Preheat frying pan and add butter and a pinch or two of salt.

Fry an egg . Salt and pepper egg to taste, then salt some more.

 Cut the donut in half. Not that way! The other way. You're making a sandwich.

Cut the cheese. Not that way! The other way. You're making a sandwich.

Add cheese, bacon, egg to the sandwich. Sprinkle with salt.

Add the top half on the donut.

Place the confectioner's sugar in your hand and make a fist. When someone is looking, pretend to scratch your head and let the sugar sprinkle down on top of the sandwich. When the person looks at you funny, tell them you

have a dandruff problem. This is the perfect technique to ensure they won't
want to eat any of your delicious donut sandwich.

Serves 1

NUTRITION AT A GLANCE

Per serving: 4200 calories, 10 g protein,
210 g carbohydrates, 199 g fat, 199 g saturated fats,
2010 mg sodium, 389 mg cholesterol, 1 g fiber

Bacon, Egg, and Cheese Bagel

An easy to make early morning treat. We've all heard that breakfast is the most important meal of the day. You may want to eat three or four of these sandwiches just to make up for some breakfasts you skipped in the past.

1 Kosher bagel

2 tablespoon butter (1 for the bagels, 1 for cooking eggs)

2 Kosher eggs

1 slice Kosher cheese

2 slices cooked bacon

Preheat skillet.

Slice bagel in half.

Butter each side and place butter side down in the skillet until toasty. Remove bagel and set aside.

Add butter to skillet. Fry the eggs.

Add eggs, bacon, and cheese to the bagel.

Serves 1

NUTRITION AT A GLANCE

Per serving: 760 calories, 21 g protein,
69 g carbohydrates, 19 g fat, 9 g saturated fats,
1405 mg sodium, 145 mg cholesterol, 2 g fiber

Cake Batter Pancakes & Ice Cream

This recipe puts the cake back into pancake. Pancakes aren't supposed to be made with oatmeal and covered in fruit. Pancakes are fried up cakes in a frying pan frosted in sugary sweetness. If your breakfast doesn't make you want to hum happy birthday, then it's not a real pancake.

1 1/2 cups all-purpose flour

2/3 cup yellow cake mix

1 tablespoon sugar

3/4 teaspoon ~~gun powder~~ baking powder

Pinch of salt

2 large eggs

1 teaspoon vanilla

1 1/2 cups whole milk (don't use 2% or low-fat milk)

1 tablespoon butter (for frying)

1 can of vanilla frosting

Colorful sprinkles

1 – 2 scoops of ice cream

Combine flour, cake mix, baking powder, sugar, and salt in a bowl and mix well.

Beat the egg, milk, and vanilla in a bowl until the batter is a little lumpy. Don't over mix. If batter is too thick, add more milk. If batter is too thin, enjoy your runny pancakes. If the batter is just right, you must be Goldilocks. Add some sprinkles to the batter.

Preheat a frying pan and add butter.

Drop the batter from a large spoon, about ¼ cup, onto frying pan. Cook until pancake is golden brown, or until surface begins to bubble. If pancake turns black or catches on fire, you cooked it too long and will need to start over. Flip and cook the other side.

In a microwave safe bowl, heat frosting until it just melts.

Pour glaze over stacks of pancakes and top with sprinkles.

Add a scoop or two of ice cream next to the pancake stack.

Serves 2 (about 12 large pancakes)

NUTRITION AT A GLANCE

Per serving: 940 calories, 12 g protein,
66 g carbohydrates, 39 g fat, 11 g saturated fats,
1020 mg sodium, 138 mg cholesterol, 0 g fiber

OOEY, GOOEY CINNAMON ROLLS

These cinnamon rolls are ooey and gooey… that's why they're called ooey, gooey cinnamon rolls. They provide an efficient way to get your entire week's supply of calories, saturated fat, and carbs in one helping.

1 cup warm whole milk

2 large eggs

1/3 cup melted butter

4 ½ cups bread flour (all-purpose flour won't work for this purpose)

1 teaspoon salt

½ cup white sugar

2 ½ teaspoons bread machine yeast

1 cup brown sugar

2 ½ tablespoons cinnamon

1/3 cup butter

3 ounces cream cheese

¼ cup butter

1 ½ cups confectioners' sugar

½ teaspoon vanilla

1/8 teaspoon salt

Dissolve the yeast in the warm milk.

In another bowl, mix the sugar, butter, salt, and eggs. Add flour and mix until smooth.

On a lightly floured surface, knead dough into a ball (about 5 minutes). Place in well-greased bowl, cover and let rise until doubled in size, about an hour. In the meantime, fold laundry, clean the dishes, mop the floor, wash your car, vacuum the house, read a book, watch a soap opera, and start making lunch.

After dough had doubled in size, roll dough out on a floured surface into a 16 by 21-inch rectangle. Spread 1/3 cup of melted butter all over dough. Mix sugar and cinnamon and sprinkle over buttered dough.

Roll up dough and cut into 12 slices. Coat the bottom of baking pan with butter. Cover and let rise until doubled in size, about 30 minutes. Meanwhile, preheat oven to 400 degrees F.

Bake cinnamon rolls until golden brown, about 15 minutes.

Meanwhile, mix cream cheese, 1/4 cup butter, confectioners' sugar, vanilla, and salt. Spread over slightly cooled rolls.

Serves 3 (makes 1 dozen)

NUTRITION AT A GLANCE

Per serving: 2100 calories, 36 g protein,
324 g carbohydrates, 73 g fat, 23 g saturated fats,
1358 mg sodium, 255 mg cholesterol, 9 g fiber

HOME MADE CHOCOLATE GLAZED DONUTS

Donuts are much more nutritious then most people realize. They contain the trifecta of nutritional goodness: trans fats, sugar, and refined flour. While it's true that donuts contain empty calories, these are all located in the hole, so just eat the donut around the hole and you'll be fine.

DONUTS (THAT'S JUST THE TITLE, NOT AN INGREDIENT. YOU'LL BE MAKING HOMEMADE DONUTS.)

>   ¾ ounce active dry yeast
>
>   ½ cup warm water
>
>   2 ¼ cups whole milk, scalded, then cooled
>
>   ¾ cup sugar
>
>   1 ½ teaspoons salt
>
>   3 large eggs
>
>   ½ cup shortening
>
>   7.52 carefully measured cups all-purpose flour
>
>   Oil for frying. I recommend cooking oil, not the kind you put in your car.

GLAZE

>   1 stick of butter (½ cup)
>
>   6 ounces of chocolate

Add yeast to warm water and stir to dissolve the yeast. Scald the milk (that's scald not scold… there's no reason to yell at your milk), and let cool. If you did yell at the milk, you may want to cool down too. Combine yeast, milk, sugar, salt, eggs, shortening and 3 cups flour.

Beat on low until the dough is smooth, about 30 seconds. Beat on medium for 2 minutes. Stir in remaining flour and mix on medium until it's incorporated.

116

Cover the bowl and let the dough rise in a warm place until doubled in size, about 30 minutes.

When ready, turn dough onto a lightly floured surface. Roll out dough to a ½ inch thickness. Cut with doughnut or cookie cutter. Cover and let rise in a warm place until doubled in size, about 30 minutes.

Make the glaze by melting the butter and chocolate until smooth.

Heat the oil to 350 degrees F. Cook on each side for about one minute. Place donuts on a cookie sheet covered with paper towels to drain.

Glaze the donuts. Optional: add sprinkles.

Serves 3 (Makes a baker's dozen. That's 13 donuts for you non-bakers)

NUTRITION AT A GLANCE

Per serving: 1330 calories, 20 g protein,
167 g carbohydrates, 53 g fat, 31 g saturated fats,
771 mg sodium, 134 mg cholesterol, 4 g fiber

LOADED MACHO NACHOS

This nacho recipe is an authentic Italian dish just like they make on the streets of Naples. Nachos aren't just for Super Bowl parties and dive bars. Nachos are also great for lunch as they have all the great toppings you love.

1 bag of corn tortilla chips

1 pound of ground beef (real beef, not the lean stuff)

1 pound can of refried beans. I know it looks and smells like dog food, but it tastes good once it's cooked.

¼ cup of water

2 cups of shredded Mexican cheese

1 white onion, finely diced

Taco seasoning packet

2 plum tomatoes

Black olives, sliced

3 green onions, chopped

2 cups sour cream (not the non-fat or low-fat crap)

1 cup guacamole

Fresh cilantro leaves

Jalapeno , optional. You can't call these Macho Nachos if you leave off the jalapeno. You'll have to refer to your nachos as Girly Nachos.

Salt & pepper to taste.

Preheat the oven to 350 degrees F. Meanwhile, sing "La Cucaracha" while spraying a cookie sheet with non-stick cooking spray.

Cook the ground beef and diced onions until beef is browned. Add the taco seasoning and water and cook until most of the water is absorbed.

Spread the tortilla chips on the cookie sheet and top with the taco beef, tomatoes, black olives, and cheese.

Bake until cheese is melted, about 6 or 7 minutes. Remove, from oven and top with green onions, cilantro, sour cream, and guacamole.

Serves 2

NUTRITION AT A GLANCE

Per serving: 2530 calories, 95 g protein,
239 g carbohydrates, 145 g fat, 92 g saturated fats,
6085 mg sodium, 244 mg cholesterol, 31 g fiber

MOCHA BREVE BREAKFAST SMOOTHIE

Wake your ass up in the morning with this delicious morning kick start. If you wake up around lunch time and need to get some instant energy, this breakfast smoothie will do the trick.

> 1 cup heavy cream
>
> 1 tablespoon peanut butter
>
> 1/8 cup of chocolate syrup
>
> 2 tablespoon sugar
>
> 1 tablespoon honey
>
> 3 shots of caffeinated espresso
>
> ½ gram uncut cocaine
>
> 1 cup ice (frozen water, not meth)

Blend in your blender until smooth and enjoy!

Serves 1

NUTRITION AT A GLANCE

Per serving: 750 calories, 5 g protein,
0.5 g cocaine, 20 g fat, 20 g saturated fats,
150 mg sodium, 10 mg cholesterol, 2 g fiber

BACON BUTTY

The funny sounding sandwich that tastes great. British scientists at Leeds University spent over 1,000 hours testing 700 variants on the traditional bacon sandwich to create a formula for the perfect bacon sandwich: $N = C + \{fb(cm) \cdot fb(tc)\} - fb(Ts) + fc \cdot ta$, where N=force in Newtons required to break the cooked bacon, fb=function of the bacon type, fc=function of the condiment/filling effect, Ts=serving temperature, tc=cooking time, ta=time or duration of application of condiment/filling, cm=cooking method, C=Newtons required to break uncooked bacon. This sandwich also makes a great hangover cure.

> 2 slices of highly-processed white bread or crusty bread roll. The butt-end of the bread loaf is fine… this is called bacon butty.
>
> 4 tablespoons of butter (1 to fry the bacon, 2 for the sandwich, and 1 to snack on as you make your sandwich)
>
> 6 slices of bacon
>
> Steak sauce (optional). Use TP Sauce if you can find it. Otherwise find a sweet, tangy steak sauce.

Bread may be toasted if you prefer. If you're running late, just bring the toaster into the shower with you.

Butter the bread, load on the fried bacon, and add desired sauce. Enjoy!

Serves 1 Nerd with a Funny Accent

NUTRITION AT A GLANCE

Per serving: 450 calories, 15 g protein,
65 g carbohydrates, 10 g fat, 2 g saturated fats,
965 mg sodium, 0 mg cholesterol, 3 g fiber

FLUFFERNUTTER

Another funny sounding sandwich that tastes great. This sandwich is so delicious that Massachusetts has tried several times to make the fluffernutter the official state sandwich.

2 slices highly-processed white bread

Peanut butter

Marshmallow Fluff

Spread peanut butter on one slice of bread, and marshmallow fluff on the other slice. Put the two slices of bread together (gooey stuff in the inside), and enjoy!

Serves 1

NUTRITION AT A GLANCE

Per serving: 300 calories, 6 g protein,
36 g carbohydrates, 13 g fat, 3 g saturated fats,
450 mg sodium, 25 mg cholesterol, 2 g fiber

FROSTING SANDWICH

You can't eat cake for lunch, but you can eat frosting sandwiches. This recipe was adapted (with some major changes) from the Vegan Tofu and Butternut Squash recipe from Vegetarian Times Magazine. I'm pretty sure this recipe is vegetarian friendly. It just wouldn't taste as good with a big slab of meat.

2 slices highly processed white bread

Frosting, any flavor

Tip: When shopping for bread, look for bread that contains preservatives, GMOs, added sugar, and artificial flavors and coloring.

Place one slice of white bread on a plate. Spread a generous amount of frosting on the slice of bread. When finished, place the second slice of bread on top. Cut in half and enjoy. This recipe is also great as an open faced sandwich. For extra nutrients, you can also butter the bread and fry this up like a grilled cheese sandwich!

Serves 1

NUTRITION AT A GLANCE

Per serving: a lot of calories, no protein,
a lot of carbohydrates, a lot of fat, a lot of sodium, no fiber,
Who reads nutritional info for a frosting sandwich?

DEEP FRIED PEANUT BUTTER & JELLY SANDWICH

Just like mom used to make, except deep fried. It also tastes a whole lot better than the sandwiches mom used to make.

2 slices highly processed white bread

Peanut Butter

Jelly

2 large eggs

½ teaspoon vanilla

1/4 cup flour

Pinch of salt.

1/4 cup whole milk

3 cups oil for frying

Lots of love

Preheat a frying pan with the oil.

Make your peanut butter and jelly sandwich.

Mix the flour and salt. Add in the milk. In another bowl, whisk the eggs and vanilla. Add the eggs to the flour mixture.

Dip your PB&J sandwich into the batter and cover completely. Add the sandwich to the frying pan. Cook until golden brown. Warning: don't deep fry your hand or fingers.

Variations: Try deep fried maple syrup and bacon sandwiches, deep fried fluffernutter sandwiches, or deep fried frosting sandwiches. Pretty much just try dry frying everything in your kitchen.

Serves 1

NUTRITION AT A GLANCE

Per serving: 635 calories, 5 g protein,
36 g carbohydrates, 100 g fat, 35 g saturated fats,
435 mg sodium, 22 mg cholesterol, 2 g fiber

CREAM CHEESE, BACON, & CARAMELIZED ONION HOT DOG

Eating this hot dog doesn't mean you've lost the will to live. It means you know how to live.

¼ pound hot dog or sausage (pork or beef, no low fat meat like turkey or armadillo)

Hot dog bun, highly-processed white flour

Full-fat cream cheese, chilled

2 slices of fried bacon (Yeah bacon!)

Caramelized-white onion

BBQ sauce

Place cooked hot dog in bun. Add cold cream cheese, fried bacon, and caramelized onions. Cover with some sweet BBQ sauce. Eat and enjoy!

Serves 1

NUTRITION AT A GLANCE

Per serving: 612 calories, 12 g protein,
24 g carbohydrates, 40 g fat, 18 g saturated fats,
911 mg sodium, 36 mg cholesterol, 1 g fiber

STROMBOLI

Take a night off from eating pizza with this tasty dinner that is essentially a rolled up pizza with a fancy name. Don't confuse this with a Zamboni which is used to clean ice rinks and doesn't taste nearly as good.

> 14 inch pizza dough ball. You can buy one from your local pizzeria or use the New York Style Pizza recipe in this book to make your dough.
>
> 1/8 pound, thinly sliced prosciutto
>
> 1/8 pound, thinly sliced pepperoni
>
> ½ cup shredded whole milk mozzarella
>
> 1/8 cup freshly grated parmesan
>
> 1 large egg, beaten

Preheat oven to 375 degrees F.

Grease a large baking sheet.

Roll out dough to 15" by 12"

Add the toppings.

Roll up jelly roll style.

Pinch the edges closed.

Cut a few slits along the top.

Brush the top of the Stromboli with beaten egg.

When you hear the smoke detector, dinner is ready!

Cool slightly before serving.

Serves 2

NUTRITION AT A GLANCE

Per serving: 1,950 calories, 90 g protein,
101 g carbohydrates, 121 g fat, 50 g saturated fats,
5,800 mg sodium, 322 mg cholesterol, 8 g fiber

LASAGNA

No diet recipe list can be complete without Garfield's favorite dish, lasagna. With its several layers of carbohydrates, full-fat mozzarella cheese, and high sodium-filled sauce, it can contain enough calories to feed a sumo wrestler.

> 1 package of lasagna noodles (1 pound)
>
> 1 pound full-fat mozzarella
>
> 1/2 pound parmesan
>
> 1 pound ricotta cheese
>
> Jar Meat Sauce. Find one with sausage, plus the store bought sauce is usually loaded with sugar.
>
> 1/2 pound spinach, rinsed and chopped
>
> Salt. Add to taste, or until you feel a heart attack coming on.

Preheat the oven to 400 degrees F.

Boil a pot of water and cook the lasagna noodles according to the directions on the package. Don't overcook, or they'll get soggy. Nobody likes a soggy noodle. Drain noodles once they are done cooking, and separate them, otherwise they can get sticky. Nobody likes a sticky noodle either. If you really messed up this recipe, you may have soggy, sticky noodles.

While the pasta is boiling, bring out the cheese. You'll probably want to buy grated cheese to avoid the exercise of grating it yourself.

Now let's make some lasagna!

Spread enough sauce to cover the bottom of a pan. Place a layer of lasagna noodles over the sauce so that they don't overlap (or least not much). Spread a generous amount of ricotta over the noodles. Then sprinkle with heaping handfuls of the other cheese. Keep building these layers. The top layer should be cheese. If you have extra cheese left over, dump it on top. You can never have too much cheese.

You should have the ½ pound spinach left. Pick it up and throw it in the trash. No one likes spinach in their lasagna! What kind of lasagna are you trying to make? First you make soggy, sticky noodles... now you try to feed us spinach?

Cover the casserole lightly with aluminum foil. Bake at 400 F for about 45 minutes or until golden brown. Remove from the oven and let sit for 10 minutes before serving.

Serves IV (4)

ROMAN NVTRITION AT A GLANCE

Per serving: MCDXL calories, LXXXIX g protein,
CI g carbohydrates, LXV g fat, XXV g saturated fats,
MMMMCMXCIX mg sodium, CCXCI mg cholesterol, XII g fiber

FETTUCCINE ALFREDO

A diet favorite. You see this recipe in all the diets books, but I'm going to include it here anyway. Known simply as "heart attack on a plate", Fettuccine Alfredo is a delicious dish of creamy decadence. The heavy, fatty, white sauce is traditionally made with cream, butter, and parmesan cheese. This is a recipe to die for! Feel free to pork out and eat as much pasta as you want. Just make sure to follow it up by eating an equal amount anti-pasta. They'll cancel each other out.

> 1 package of fettuccine noodles (1 pound)
>
> 2 sticks of butter (1 cup). Anything made with 2 sticks of butter is going to taste delicious!
>
> 1 cup heavy whipping cream
>
> 1 ½ cups freshly shredded parmesan cheese
>
> 1 teaspoon salt

Cook the fettuccine noodles according to the direction on the package.

If you were lazy and just bought a jar of pre-made Alfredo sauce, dump it in the noodles, stir, and you're done. Otherwise, keep reading.

While the noodles are cooking, grab a sauce pan and heat the butter and whipping cream over low heat until melted. Stir in cheese and salt. Dump it in the noodles, stir, and you're done.

Warning: While eating Fettuccine Alfredo, if you experience chest pain or tightness, shortness of breath, dizziness, sweating, nausea, and your left arm goes numb, call 911

Serves 2

NUTRITION AT A GLANCE

Per serving: 14,565 calories, 46 g protein,
845 g carbohydrates, 509 g fat, 209 g saturated fats,
2,082 mg sodium, 484 mg cholesterol, 8 g fiber

DOUBLE BACON, DOUBLE CHEESE, DOUBLE MAYO, DOUBLE BURGER

This is the food you eat right before you start a diet. Double bypass surgery between the buns. Remember to always practice safe eating. Always use condiments. And make sure to drink a diet soda with this.

This recipe was inspired from the following idea of a diet. You order a bacon cheese burger with extra bacon, but hold the extra bacon.

Two ¼ pound All Beef Hamburger Patties

White Bun

Blue Cheese

2 Thick Slices of Bacon

1 - 2 Tablespoons Mayonnaise. You may substitute Baconnaise.

I think you can figure this one out on your own. If not, go to a drive through and order a double bacon cheeseburger.

Serves 1

NUTRITION AT A GLANCE

Per serving: 701 calories, 52 g protein,
39 g carbohydrates, 42 g fat, 12 g saturated fats,
1,605 mg sodium, 165 mg cholesterol, 1 g fiber

NEW YORK STYLE PIZZA

Fitness? No, more like fit this whole pizza in my mouth. I tried running, but I kept dropping my pizza. Does running out of pizza count as cardio?

Bread flour, 12.0 ounces

Warm Water, 7.5 ounces

Active Dry Yeast, 0.06 ounce

Salt, 0.18 ounces

Olive Oil, 0.12 ounces

Tomato Sauce, 10 ounce can

Mozzarella Cheese, one pound

Toppings (Your Choice)

Add water and salt to a mixing bowl. Mix on low as you slowly add the flour and then the yeast. Increase speed to medium until all the flour is picked up. Lower the speed to low and add the oil. Increase speed back to medium for about 10 minutes.

Roll dough into a ball and place it in a lightly oiled bowl. Place uncovered in the refrigerator for two hours. After two hours, cover the bowl and allow the dough to sit in the refrigerator overnight.

The next day, remove dough from refrigerator and allow it to sit at room temperature for two hours. In the meantime, preheat oven as hot as possible (400 degrees F +). Use a large pizza stone if you have one for best results.

Form dough into a 16 inch pizza skin. Cover with tomato sauce, cheese, and desired toppings. Add pizza to oven until cheese is melted. If crust browns faster than the top, try heating pizza on broil for a minute or so.

If you cook the pizza too long, don't worry you just burned over 1,500 calories in under 30 minutes. Plus, if dinner sucks you can always order a pizza.

Serves 2 (or 1 if you consider this a personal size pizza)

NUTRITION AT A GLANCE

Per serving: 1,620 calories, 80 g protein,
118 g carbohydrates, 73 g fat, 21 g saturated fats,
3,645 mg sodium, 171 mg cholesterol, 3.14159 g fiber (it's pizza pie)

SAGE-BUTTER GNOCCHI

This is the perfect meal to make at home. That way you can avoid the awkwardness of trying to pronounce "gnocchi" in front of the waiter.

2 (12 ounce) packages potato gnocchi

½ stick of butter (it doesn't matter which half)

1 clove garlic, minced

1 teaspoon dried sage

1/4 teaspoon salt

1/4 cup grated Parmesan cheese

Add gnocchi to a large pot of boiling water. Once the gnocchi floats to the top (2-3 minutes), remove and drain. Normally, I don't eat floaters, but I make an exception for gnocchi.

Add butter and garlic to a frying pan. After 5 minutes, add the sage and salt. Mix in the gnocchi and then top with cheese.

Serves 2

NUTRITION AT A GLANCE

Per serving: 770 calories, 17 g protein,
65 g carbohydrates, 55 g fat, 12 g saturated fats,
1,000 mg sodium, 150 mg cholesterol, 5 g fiber

MAGGIE'S BIG ASS BURRITO

Maggie's Big Ass Burrito recipe is named after my aunt. However, she never really liked it when I called her big ass.

This is a great dinner to have along with a bag or two of tortilla chips. It will probably also give you explosive diarrhea, but don't let that stop you. This burrito is worth it!

1 extra-large flour tortilla

½ cup pork carnitas (cooked)

¼ cup Mexican rice (cooked)

¼ cup pinto beans (cooked)

¼ cup cheddar cheese

4 tablespoons salsa

1 tablespoon guacamole

2 tablespoons full-fat sour cream

Add the pork, rice, beans, and cheese to your tortilla. Fold up the burrito. Add the burrito to a frying plan on medium heat. Lightly brown each side of the burrito. Top the burrito with the salsa, guacamole, and sour cream.

Serves Uno

NUTRITION AT A GLANCE

Per serving: 600 calories, 30 g protein,
65 g carbohydrates, 25 g fat, 5 g saturated fats,
911 mg sodium, 80 mg cholesterol, 5 g fiber

TWICE BAKED POTATO

These aren't those disgusting broccoli and cheese baked potatoes that everyone hates. These twice baked potatoes are loaded with bacon, cheese, salt, butter, and sour cream!

> 6 large russet potatoes
>
> 3 green onions sliced
>
> Salt
>
> 6 strips bacon, more if you eat the bacon while cooking, cooked and crumbled
>
> 6 tablespoons sour cream
>
> 1/4 cup whole milk
>
> 4 tablespoons butter
>
> 6 ounces cheddar cheese grated. I usually give mine an A+.

Preheat oven to 400 degrees F. Stab each potato with a fork. There is no reason to do this in preparing the food, but it is fun. Bake the potatoes for an hour.

Optional Lazy Person Directions: Microwave potatoes on High until soft, then toss them in the oven for about 20 minutes.

Once you remove the potatoes from the oven, let them cool for about 10 minutes so you don't burn your fingers. Cut the potatoes lengthwise. Scoop out the insides into a bowl. Add sour cream, butter, milk, half of the cheese, half the green onions, and half the bacon. Add salt to taste. When in doubt, add more salt.

Scoop the filling back into the potato skins. Top with the other half of the cheese, green onions, and bacon. Bake another 20 minutes. If the potatoes catch on fire during baking or come out burned, try reducing the oven temperature next time. I've actually never made this recipe as I order twice baked potatoes at restaurants and bars because I don't cook. I probably should have disclosed that earlier. Bon appetit!

Serves 2 as far as I know

NUTRITION AT A GLANCE

Per serving: 2,500 calories, 60 g protein,
180 g carbohydrates, 180 g fat, 70 g saturated fats,
3,200 mg sodium, 370 mg cholesterol, 15 g fiber

THREE CHEESE & BACON MACARONI AND CHEESE

If you're trying to avoid fried food, you'll be happy to hear that mac & cheese is baked! If you don't mind fried food, use the left overs to make grilled macaroni and cheese sandwiches. Try it.

1 pound elbow macaroni (the same stuff kids use to make macaroni art)

6 slices bacon, cooked and crumbled

8 tablespoons butter

6 tablespoons all-purpose flour

1/4 teaspoon salt

1 teaspoon black pepper

3 cups whole milk

1 cup heavy cream

1 pound shredded sharp cheddar cheese

4 oz. shredded provolone cheese

4 oz. shredded asiago cheese

2 cups panko bread crumbs

Preheat oven to 325 degrees F.

Cook macaroni according to package directions. Drain.

In a large sauce pan melt butter.

Whisk in flour until smooth.

Add milk and whisk until thickened, about 5 minutes.

Whisk in salt, pepper (careful with the pepper, otherwise you'll get macaroni and sneeze), heavy cream, and cheese until melted.

Stir in the bacon and macaroni.

In a separate pan, melt 2 tablespoons of butter and mix in bread crumbs until the butter is absorbed. Set aside.

Spoon macaroni mixture into a lightly greased 13x9 baking dish. Top with bread crumbs. Bake for 3 hours. Just kidding… just bake it until golden brown, around 12 to 15 minutes.

Serves 3

NUTRITION AT A GLANCE

Per serving: 1,500 calories, 70 g protein,
150 g carbohydrates, 70 g fat, 50 g saturated fats,
2,000 mg sodium, 200 mg cholesterol, 6 g fiber

LOADED PUB WAFFLE FRIES

Extra fries sounds a lot like exercise.

Why eat regular fries when you can eat fancy fries in the shape of waffles smothered with gooey cheese and bacon and sour cream. Everyone loves pub food.

> 4 cups waffle fries
>
> 1 teaspoon steak seasoning
>
> 1 cup shredded cheddar cheese
>
> 2 tablespoons chopped green onions
>
> 2 tablespoons bacon bits
>
> Sour cream (for garnish)

Preheat oven to 450 degrees F. Obviously it's F, not C. The only way you'd get your oven that hot is on self-cleaning mode.

Pour out waffle fries onto a cookie sheet. Bake for 25 minutes.

Remove fries and sprinkle with steak seasoning. Mound fries with bacon bits, onions, and cheese. If you don't have a cheese shredder, you can always use the screen door.

Bake for another 3 minutes to melt cheese. Remove from oven, top with sour cream.

Serves 2

NUTRITION AT A GLANCE

Per serving: 1,650 calories, 70 g protein,
125 g carbohydrates, 100 g fat, 20 g saturated fats,
4,000 mg sodium, 210 mg cholesterol, 9 g fiber

CREAM OF TOMATO GORGONZOLA SOUP

Just like the last recipe… why would you want a boring bowl of tomato soup? Add some spices and fatty food to it to give it some taste. That's what I'm talking about. This recipe pairs well with a glass of Alka-Seltzer.

1 (26 ounce) can of your finest tomato soup

2 (14.5 ounce) cans Italian-style diced tomatoes, undrained

1/2 cup water

1 cup whole milk or cream

4 ounces crumbled gorgonzola cheese

2 tablespoons minced garlic

1 tablespoon dried basil

1 teaspoon onion powder

Combine the tomato soup, diced tomatoes, water, and milk in a large saucepan over medium heat. Stir until lukewarm, or how ever hot you like your soup. Then stir in gorgonzola cheese, garlic, basil, and onion powder. Reduce heat to low; simmer 15 to 20 minutes, stirring often.

Serves 2

NUTRITION AT A GLANCE

Per serving: 500 calories, 25 g protein (aka dead fly),
52 g carbohydrates, 20 g fat, 12 g saturated fats,
2,300 mg sodium, 80 mg cholesterol, 7 g fiber

BACON FETA BEANS

This is the closest thing to eating veggies you're going to get on the Contrarian Diet. Personally, when I make this recipe I just eat around the beans. It's not wasteful.

> 8 slices bacon - cooked, crumbled and divided
>
> 1 can of green beans (optional – this recipe is delicious without the beans)
>
> 1 teaspoon minced garlic
>
> 4 ounces crumbled feta cheese, divided
>
> 1/2 teaspoon onion powder
>
> 1/8 teaspoon ground black pepper
>
> 2 tablespoons water

Place bacon in a large, deep skillet. Cook over medium high heat until evenly browned but only slightly crisp. Drain grease, leaving a small amount in the skillet for later use. Crumble bacon, reserving 2 tablespoons for garnish, and set aside.

Open can of green beans. If you slice your fingertip on the rim of the can, clean up blood. Actually, let's just make this a little safer and use a 16 ounce bag of frozen beans. Dump the frozen beans into a microwave safe bowl. Cover and cook for about 3 minutes until the edges are scalding hot and the middle is still frozen. When beans are thawed, drain the liquid, pat dry, and set aside.

Reheat skillet with residual bacon grease over medium-high heat. Stir in bacon and garlic until garlic is lightly golden. Add green beans and feta cheese, and season with onion powder and black pepper. Cook and stir until most of the feta cheese has melted, about 2 minutes. Transfer to a serving dish, and garnish with remaining feta cheese and crumbled bacon. Serve hot.

Serves 2

NUTRITION AT A GLANCE

Per serving: 330 calories, 25 g protein,
18 g carbohydrates, 25 g fat, 10 g saturated fats,
1,500 mg sodium, 85 mg cholesterol, 6 g fiber

AUTHENTIC IRISH GARLIC MASHED POTATOES

This is an authentic Irish recipe straight from the IRA field manual recipe section. These are the official mashed potatoes that the Irish use for food fights.

This is also part of the garlic diet. The diet works like this. You eat a lot of garlic because you look thinner from a distance.

> 5 pounds Yukon Gold potatoes. Don't ask me why the recipe uses northwestern Canadian potatoes instead of Irish potatoes.
>
> 4 cloves garlic, crushed.
>
> 3/4 cups butter
>
> 1 package (8 Oz.) cream cheese, softened
>
> 3/4 cup half-and-half
>
> 1 teaspoon salt

The first step is interrogating the potato. Grab a potato. Tell it to talk. If it doesn't immediately respond, place it under running water. Repeat a couple times.

If the potato remains silent, look the potato right in the eyes. If it doesn't talk, cut its eyes out Wait a few seconds. If it still doesn't talk, start peeling off its skin. If it hasn't talked by the time all its skin is removed, bring the potato over to the stove.

Start boiling a large pot of water. Warn the potato if it doesn't start talking, you're going to throw it and his other potato friends into the pot of boiling water.

If the potato is still silent, take out a large knife. Slowly cut the potato in half lengthwise. Still nothing? Cut the potato in half again.

Give the potato one more chance to talk. If it doesn't, throw it into the boiling water for 30 minutes. Then ask the potato to talk. If you don't get a response, stab the potato with a fork. The fork should easily slide into the potato. If not, keep boiling it.

If this potato hasn't talked by this point, you're going to need to take a different approach. Drain the water. Let the potato sit in the pot and try buttering it up. Use the full ¾ cup of butter if you need to. Make those potatoes happy. Give them garlic, cream cheese, half-and-half, and salt. Just don't allow them to escape.

Politely ask the potato one more time to talk. If it refuses, violently mash the potato until it becomes a creamy mush. Then eat it.

Serves 5

NUTRITION AT A GLANCE

Per serving: 475 calories, 9 g protein,
68 g carbohydrates, 20 g fat, 9 g saturated fats,
260 mg sodium, 48 mg cholesterol, 9 g fiber

SNICKERS SALAD

If you normally snicker and shake your head no when someone asks if you want some salad, then this salad is for you. If you've been trying to cut back on greens, you'll enjoy this salad.

 1 (8 ounce) package cream cheese, softened

 1 cup powdered sugar

 1 (12 ounce) container whip cream, thawed

 6 Snickers candy bars, cut into ½ inch pieces

 4 - 5 granny smith apples, cored and cut into bite sized pieces

In a large bowl, mix cream cheese and powdered sugar. Fold in whip cream. Fold in apples and Snickers bars. Refrigerate until serving.

Serves 3

NUTRITION AT A GLANCE

Per serving: 880 calories, 10 g protein,
31 g carbohydrates, 40 g fat, 25 g saturated fats,
700 mg sodium, 25 mg cholesterol, 8 g fiber

Drinks

TWINKIE MILKSHAKE

The recipe below is adapted from The Twinkies Cookbook, but with more sugar and more fat. You really can have your Twinkie and drink it too... along with 37 highly processed ingredients, 9 teaspoons of sugar, high fructose corn syrup, hydrogenated oils, artificial colors, and other chemical additives.

2 Twinkies

1 pint chocolate ice cream

½ cup white sugar

1 cup heavy cream

Whipped cream, for topping

Maraschino cherry, for topping

Blend the Twinkies, ice cream, sugar and cream until smooth. Pour into a glass and top with whip cream and a maraschino cherry.

Serves 1

NUTRITION AT A GLANCE

Per serving: a week's worth of calories, ? g protein,
? g carbohydrates, a ton of fat, ? g saturated fats,
? mg sodium, ? mg cholesterol, ? g fiber
(You're seriously looking at nutritional information for a Twinkie
Milkshake?)

148

IRISH COFFEE

"Only Irish coffee provides in a single glass all four essential food groups: alcohol, caffeine, sugar and fat" Alex Levin.

It doesn't need to be St. Patrick's Day to enjoy a good Irish coffee.

     1 cup hot brewed coffee

     1 tablespoon brown sugar

     1 jigger Irish whiskey

     1 jigger Irish cream liqueur

     1 tablespoon Heavy cream, whipped

A jigger is pretty much as much booze as you it to be. If you're the type of person that has to measure it out, just use 1 1/2 ounces or 3 tablespoons.

Pour coffee into a mug. Stir in brown sugar, whiskey, and liqueur. Top drink with whipped heavy cream. I like to drink my Irish coffee in the morning while eating a bowl of Lucky Charms.

Serves 1

MUDSLIDE

Losing weight is a constant battle many of us fight throughout our lives. Lucky for me, I'm a lover not a fighter. I love mudslides. Dieting is also a constant battle between my love for food and not wanting to get fat. That's why I stick to liquid diets, like Mudslides.

2 ounces Baileys Irish Cream

1 ounce Kahlua coffee liqueur

2 cups vanilla ice cream

Chocolate syrup

Whipped cream

Blend Baileys, Kahlua, and ice cream. Pour chocolate syrup around the inside of a glass. Pour contents of blender into glass. Top with whip cream and more chocolate syrup.

Serves 1

BLOODY MARY

Your doctor said it was OK for you to drink Bloody Marys for breakfast. He didn't say that in those exact words. He said you need to reduce the stress in your life, which is pretty much the same thing.

1 1/2 ounces vodka

3 ounces tomato juice. You say tomato. I say Bloody Mary.

1 lemon juice

1 dash Worcestershire sauce

3 dashes Tabasco sauce

1 pinch pepper

1 pinch salt

1/4 teaspoon celery salt

2 tsp horseradish

1 stick celery (for garnish)

Lemon or lime wedge (for garnish)

I know there are a lot of dashes of this and pinches of that in this recipe. It sounds like you're making a witch's potion, but trust me you're just making a drink. Put on a tall, black, pointy hat, and stir all ingredients together while cackling. Pour into a glass filled with ice. Garnish with lemon or lime wedge and celery stick, or just toss the fruit and veggies in the garbage where they belong.

Serves 1

MIMOSA

A great way to start the day before heading to work. Alcohol doesn't make you fat; it makes you lean... against tables, chairs, walls, and ugly people. Recipe difficulty: Hard.

>   3 ounces orange juice

>   3 ounces Champagne

Fill champagne flute (or coffee mug if you're heading to work) half full of champagne. Fill the rest of the glass with orange juice. This is one of those recipes where you may lose weight and your driver's license.

Serves 1

LONG ISLAND ICE TEA

As many calories as a McDonald's Big Mac. I have a friend that's on the Long Island Ice Tea Diet. So far she's lost three days. She's also gained a terrible headache, a couple STDs, and a bunch of embarrassing photos.

> 1 ounce vodka
>
> 1 ounce tequila
>
> 1 ounce rum
>
> 1 ounce gin
>
> 1 ounce triple sec
>
> 1 1/2 ounces sweet and sour mix
>
> 1 splash cola
>
> Lemon wedge (garnish)

Add ingredients into a cocktail mixer. Shake and pour into a glass full of ice. If you don't have ice, you can substitute frozen water. Garnish with lemon wedge.

Serves 1

PEANUT BUTTER CUP MILK SHAKE

If you ever get the urge to sit down, grab a spoon, and eat an entire pint of ice cream, but you just feel too guilty doing so… then just make this milk shake instead.

> 1 pint of chocolate ice cream
>
> 1/3 cup whole milk and nothing but the milk
>
> 3 heaping tablespoons peanut butter
>
> Whipped cream (to top milkshake…and to squirt directly into your mouth when no one is looking)

Blend ingredients until creamy. Pour into glass. Top with whipped cream. Drink and repeat.

Serves 1

CHOCOLATE SHEET CAKE

I just like saying "chocolate sheet." It tastes a lot better than it sounds.

2 cups sugar

2 cups all-purpose flour

2 sticks of butter

4 tablespoons cocoa

1 cup water, or whatever you have on tap

1/2 cup buttermilk

2 large eggs, lightly beaten

1 teaspoon baking soda

1 teaspoon vanilla

Chocolate Icing

Preheat oven to 375 degrees F.

Bring butter , cocoa, water, and buttermilk to a boil in a medium saucepan, stirring constantly, until butter and shortening melt. Remove from heat, and mix in flour, sugar, eggs, baking soda, and vanilla.

Pour into a greased 15- x 10 x 2-inch jelly roll pan.

Bake for 20 minutes. Spread warm cake with chocolate Icing, and then eat that sheet. That's some good tasting sheet!

Serves 5

NUTRITION AT A GLANCE

Per serving: 1,400 calories, 12 g protein,
200 g carbohydrates, 60 g fat, 40 g saturated fats,
1,200 mg sodium, 100 mg cholesterol, 5 g fiber

BROWNIE SUNDAE TOPPED WITH MARASCHINO CHERRY

Everyone loves ice cream. It's full of sugar, loaded with trans fats, and artificial colors and flavors. Then top it off with some yummy maraschino cherries. That will add some processed fruit packed with sugar and artificial colors like red-40 and red-3 dyes.

    1 large brownie

    2 – 3 scoops vanilla ice cream

    Chocolate sauce

    Whipped cream

    Maraschino cherry (or a crouton if you want to think of this as a salad)

Make a sundae out of the ingredients above.

Serves 1

NUTRITION AT A GLANCE

Per serving: 600 calories, 8 g protein,
60 g carbohydrates, 20 g fat, 15 g saturated fats,
300 mg sodium, 30 mg cholesterol, 3 g fiber

FUDGE

If there's chocolate spread all over this page, someone may have fudged this recipe.

2 3/4 cups sugar

4 ounces unsweetened chocolate (this is a diet recipe… actually, you'll be adding a lot of sugar, so don't worry)

3 tablespoons butter, plus more for greasing pan

1 cup half-and-half

1 tablespoon corn syrup

1 tablespoon vanilla extract

1 cup chopped nuts, like almonds, walnuts, or pecans.

Grease an 8 by 8-inch pan with butter.

Combine, sugar, chocolate, 1 1/2 tablespoons of the butter, half and half, and corn syrup.

Cook over medium heat, stirring constantly, until chocolate boils.

Add a candy thermometer and boil until mixture reaches 234 degrees F. Don't eat the candy thermometer – it's not actually made out of candy.

Remove from the heat. Add remaining butter and vanilla. Do not stir. Let the mixture cool to around 120 degrees F (about 10 minutes).

Optional: Add nuts and mix.

Beat fudge with wooden spoon until fudge becomes matte (about 5 minutes).

Spread into the prepared pan and let cool.

Cut into small pieces (you can eat numerous pieces at once). Store in an airtight container or just eat them all and don't worry about storing them.

Serves 1 or 2

NUTRITION AT A GLANCE

Per serving:
1,000,000 calories,
1,000,000 g fat

CHOCOLATE CHIP COOKIES

Nothing is more upsetting than mistaking an oatmeal raison cookie for a chocolate chip cookie. The only sure what to avoid oatmeal raison cookies is to bake your own chocolate chip cookies.

    1 cup butter, softened

    1 cup white sugar

    1 cup packed brown sugar

    1 teaspoon vanilla extract

    1/2 teaspoon salt

    1 teaspoon baking powder

    1 teaspoon baking soda

2 eggs

    2 cups all-purpose flour

    2-1/2 cups rolled oats, blended to powder.

    2 cups raisins… just joking, 2 cups semisweet chocolate chips

    1/4 pound finely grated chocolate bar

    2 cups chopped walnuts

Preheat oven to 350 degrees F.

Mix butter, sugars, eggs, and vanilla.

In a separate bowl, mix salt, baking powder, baking soda, flour and oatmeal.

Combine both bowls and mix.

Stir in chocolate chips, grated chocolate bar, and chopped nuts.

If you're thinking about eating the raw cookie dough, go ahead. The odds of the eggs being infected with Salmonella bacteria is only about 1 in 20,000.

Scoop one inch cookie dough balls on to greased cookie sheet. Leave 2 inches between dough. Bake for 8 -10 minutes.

Serves 5 (10 – 12 cookies per serving)

NUTRITION AT A GLANCE

Per serving: 1,500 calories, 20 g protein,
200 g carbohydrates, 80 g fat, 55 g saturated fats,
750 mg sodium, 170 mg cholesterol, 10 g fiber

BANANAS FOSTER

This is a crowd pleaser. Bananas Foster is the perfect excuse to intentionally catch something on fire in the kitchen. And it tastes great too.

1 stick salted butter

1 cup packed dark brown sugar

1/2 cup heavy cream

2 bananas, peeled and sliced. People in South America use two banana peels as a pair of slippers.

1/2 cup chopped walnuts or pecans

1/2 cup dark rum – it's for the recipe, so don't drink it.

Dash of cinnamon

Vanilla ice cream, for serving – not eating while you make the recipe.

Fire extinguisher (just in case)

Combine the butter, sugar, and cinnamon in a skillet on medium heat until butter melts.

Add cream and stir. Add banana slices and nuts.

Stir in the rum. Light rum on fire and let burn until it goes out.

Check to see if you still have eyebrows.

Spoon warm sauce over ice cream.

Serves 2

NUTRITION AT A GLANCE

Per serving: 1,050 calories, 10 g protein,
150 g carbohydrates, 50 g fat, 35 g saturated fats,
300 mg sodium, 120 mg cholesterol, 7 g fiber

CHOCOLATE CHEESECAKE

No comment.

1 ½ cups Oreo Cookies, crushed. This will take about 30 cookies (that's just the way the cookie crumbles)

2 tablespoons butter or margarine, melted

24 oz. Cream Cheese, at room temperature as long as your room temperature happens to be around 70 degrees F.

1 cup sugar

1 teaspoon vanilla extract

8 ounces chocolate chips, melted and cooled

3 large eggs

1 pair sunglasses

Preheat oven to 325 degrees F.

You actually only need about 20 cookies for 1 ½ cups. I figured you eat about 10 of them before getting to this point in the recipe. Crush the remaining 20 cookies and mix them with the melted butter. Press onto bottom of 9-inch pan. Bake 10 minutes.

Beat cream cheese, sugar and vanilla with mixer at low speed until creamy. Add chocolate, and then add eggs one at a time until blended. Pour mixture into crust.

Bake until center is almost set, about 50 minutes. I don't know how you're going to know when it's almost set, but if it does set then you know you cooked it too long. Remove from oven. Place sunglasses on top of cheesecake (now your cheesecake is completely cool). Cover pan and refrigerate cheesecake four hours or overnight… or just dig in and eat it. I don't really care, it's your cheesecake.

Serves 5

NUTRITION AT A GLANCE

Per serving: 1,000 calories, 15 g protein,
100 g carbohydrates, 75 g fat, 40 g saturated fats,
800 mg sodium, 300 mg cholesterol, 7 g fiber

MOLTEN CHOCOLATE CAKE

Molten Chocolate Cake, also known as Lava Cake, is the perfect ending to a meal. It's also world's second most dangerous cake for women. Wedding cake being the first.

> 4 ounces chocolate chips
>
> 1 stick of butter (1/2 cup)
>
> 1 cup powdered sugar
>
> 2 large eggs, unfertilized
>
> 2 egg yolks
>
> 6 tablespoon all-purpose flour
>
> 1/2 cup whipped cream

Preheat oven to 425 degrees F.

Butter bottoms and sides of four custard cups.

In a saucepan, melt chocolate chips and butter over low heat, stirring frequently. Stir in sugar. Add eggs-actly two whole eggs and egg yolks; mix well. Stir in flour. Spoon into prepared cups. Place on baking sheet.

Bake until sides are firm but centers are still soft, about 12 to 14 minutes. Let cool for one minute. Run knife or small spatula around cakes to loosen. Place plate over each cup and turn upside down so cake drops onto plate. Serve warm topped with whipped cream.

In the unlikely event that any of the eggs were fertilized, just throw the chicks into the lava cake.

Serves 2 (2 cakes per serving)

NUTRITION AT A GLANCE

Per serving: 600 calories, 16 g protein,
120 g carbohydrates, 80 g fat, 50 g saturated fats,
450 mg sodium, 500 mg cholesterol, 3 g fiber

HOMEMADE POTATO CHIPS

You probably thought air was free. Not when you buy a bag of potato chips. It's best to just make your own. Plus, you can combat the stereotype that potato chip eaters are lazy. You're not lazy if you go to the work of making your very own homemade potato chips.

1 Yukon Gold potato

Vegetable oil, for frying

Salt

Wash potato.

Fill a bowl with cold water.

Use a vegetable peeler to slice potato into chips. Place the chips into the bowl of cold water as you slice them.

Heat oil to 400 degrees F. Lower chips into the oil.

When chips are golden and crispy, remove with a slotted spoon.

Add salt.

Serves 1

NUTRITION AT A GLANCE

Per serving: 320 calories, 5 g protein,
45 g carbohydrates, 14 g fat, 10 g saturated fats,
1,200 mg sodium, 0 mg cholesterol, 4 g fiber

SOFT PRETZELS

Pretzels go great with mustard and a beer. If you want to be cool, make pretzel rods, bite the end off, and pretend you're smoking a cigar.

2 teaspoons active dry yeast

1/2 teaspoon white sugar

2 1/2 cups all-purpose flour. This ingredient can also be used as a powdered sugar substitute, simple toothpaste, laundry detergent, fake snow, artificial dandruff, and many other things since it's ALL-purpose flour.

1/4 cup white sugar

3/4 teaspoons salt

1/2 tablespoon vegetable oil

1/4 cup baking soda

Coarse salt, of course, for topping

In a small bowl, dissolve 1 teaspoon sugar and yeast in 1 1/4 cup warm water (110 degrees F). Let stand until creamy, about 5 minutes.

In a large bowl, whisk together flour, 1/2 cup sugar, and salt. Add the oil and yeast mixture and mix until it forms into dough. Knead the dough until smooth, about 8 minutes.

Return the dough to the bowl. Cover with plastic wrap and let rise in a warm place until doubled in size, about 1 hour.

Preheat oven to 450 degrees F. Grease a baking sheet.

In a large bowl, dissolve baking soda in 4 cups hot water; set aside.

Cut dough into 6 equal pieces. Roll each piece into a rope. Twist rope into a pretzel shape. Place pretzels onto the baking sheet.

Bring a pot of water to a boil. Place each pretzel in the boiling water for about 1 minute. Using tongs, pick up pretzels and place them back on the baking sheet. Sprinkle pretzels with salt.

Bake until golden brown in color, about 8 minutes.

Serves 3 (2 pretzels per serving)

NUTRITION AT A GLANCE

Per serving: 480 calories, 11 g protein,
100 g carbohydrates, 4 g fat, 2 g saturated fats,
5000 mg sodium, 0 mg cholesterol, 3 g fiber

CHOCOLATE POPCORN

Popcorn is a lot easier to make than other meals, like pea soup. Anyone can make popcorn, but no one can pea soup.

Popcorn

Chocolate If you're out of chocolate, any brown substance will do.

Make a bag of popcorn per the directions. Don't burn the popcorn! Add popcorn to a large bowl.

Place large sheet of parchment paper on the counter.

Melt chocolate... or whatever you're coating with popcorn with. Stir popcorn as you pour chocolate over the popcorn. Coat popcorn completely.

Pour chocolate popcorn onto parchment paper and allow it to cool.

Serves 1

NUTRITION AT A GLANCE

Per serving: Depends how much you make.

CHURCH STAINED GLASS WINDOWS

Usually it's a good idea to avoid chocolate, because it makes your clothes shrink. These, however, are worth it.

1 stick of butter (1/2 cup)

1 (12 ounce) package semisweet chocolate chips. I recommend semi-sweet because I know you're watching your weight.

1 (10.5 ounce) package rainbow colored miniature marshmallows

Melt chocolate chips and butter in a pan on low heat or in the microwave. Once melted, let it cool slightly and then fold in the marshmallows.

Spoon the mixture onto wax paper to form to logs. Refrigerate until logs are cool. Cut into ½ inch slices and eat! If you're going to eat an entire log by yourself in one sitting, then no need to slice. Pick it up and eat it like a banana.

Serves 2 (one log per serving)

NUTRITION AT A GLANCE

Per serving: 3,000 calories, 5 g protein,
325 g carbohydrates, 195 g fat, 50 g saturated fats,
1,000 mg sodium, 125 mg cholesterol, 25 g fiber

Peanut Butter Balls (Redacted Copy)

The perfect recipe for the new gourmet cook. Many French cooks start out by making peanut butter balls. The secret to making these peanut butter balls is XXXXXXXXXXXXXXXXXXXXXXXXXXXXXXXXX.

1/2 cup peanut butter

1/2 cup honey

XXXXXXXXXXXXXXXXXXXXXXXXX

1 cup powdered milk

XXXXXXXXXXXX XXXXXXXXXXXX

In a large bowl combine peanut butter, honey, milk, and the secret ingredients. Form the mixture into balls about the size of a peanut butter ball. Place on waxed paper and refrigerate for 20 minutes. Burn this recipe after reading.

Alternatives: You can roll the peanut butter balls in powdered sugar, crushed nuts, crushed cereal, or dip them in chocolate.

Serves 3 (4 peanut butter balls per serving)

NUTRITION AT A GLANCE

Per serving: 640 calories, 12 g protein,
72 g carbohydrates, X g fat, 38 g saturated fats,
310 mg sodium, 20 mg cholesterol, 4 g fiber

PEPPERONI PIZZA BITES

I know pepperoni pizza bites are processed food. But I gave up on eating natural foods once I learned that 80% of people die from natural causes.

4 mini bagels

3 tablespoons tomato sauce

¼ cup mozzarella cheese

8 slices of pepperoni

Slice mini bagels in half and then place on a microwave safe plate. Spread tomato sauce evenly over the top of the bagels. Top with cheese and pepperoni. Microwave until cheese is melted. It may not be gourmet, but it's faster than pizza delivery.

Serves 45 (in order to keep the nutritional information diet-appropriate)

NUTRITION AT A GLANCE

Per serving: 10 calories, 1 g protein,
2 g carbohydrates, 1 g fat, 1 g saturated fats,
40 mg sodium, 1 mg cholesterol, 0 g fiber

Brownie Ice Cream Sandwich

Warning: The following recipe is highly addictive and could be hazardous to your health. In consideration of being permitted to make the Brownie Ice Cream Sandwich recipe (hereinafter referred to as "Recipe"), I hereby release the author and publisher from any and all liability, claims, demands, or action that I may have for injuries, addictions, or sudden death out of my participation in making the Recipe or eating the ice cream sandwiches produced by following the Recipe. I understand that making this Recipe is inherently dangerous and addictive and I expressly and voluntarily assume all risk of death or personal injury sustained while making the Recipe.

Before attempting to make the Recipe, please sign below to waive your rights

_____

Signature

    2 Brownies

    1 large scoop of vanilla ice cream

    Chocolate chips or sprinkles

Place scoop of ice cream between two brownies. You can use pre-made brownies (recommended) or make your own. Roll side of sandwich with chocolate chips or chocolate sprinkles.

How to make homemade brownies: You'll need a brown piece of paper, a pencil, and scissors. Draw the letter "E" several times on the brown paper. Cut them out with the scissors.

Serves 1

NUTRITION AT A GLANCE

Per serving: 550 calories, 10 g protein,
70 g carbohydrates, 30 g fat, 18 g saturated fats,
350 mg sodium, 40 mg cholesterol,
3 g fiber (more if you made your own brownies)

CREDITS

The Cinnamon Roll French Toast recipe used with permission of Jean-Pierre's Gourmet Bakery, Paris, France.

The Frosting Sandwich recipe was adapted from the recipe used with permission of the Executive Chef at San Quentin State Prison. Basically, I added the frosting ingredient to their recipe that consisted of bread. They recommended pairing their recipe with a glass of water.

The Loaded Macho Nachos recipe was copied off the wall in the ladies restroom at Taco Bell.

Maggie's Big Ass Burrito recipe used with permission of my Aunt Maggie's big ass.

The Pepperoni Pizza Bites recipe was used with permission of the 40 year old guy next door that lives in his mother's basement.

GLOSSARY

Balanced Diet	A cookie in each hand.
Calorie	Not a unit of energy, but rather a unit of taste.
Calories	Tiny creatures that live in your closet and come out at night and sew your clothes tighter.
Cannibal	Someone who is fed up with people.
Desserter	A person who has abandoned their diet.
Diet	1) A weigh of life, 2) When you have to go to some length to change your width, 3) Did I Eat That, 4) An invented word because all the other 4-letter words were taken.
Dieting	1) Wishful shrinking. 2) Breaking the pound barrier, 3) Eating within your seams.
Eating Disorder	When you eat dis order of cheeseburgers, dis order of French fries, and dis order of soda.
Exercise	Wasted energy.
Fat	Fat is a means of storing energy in our body. It's kind of like a bank account. Don't worry about getting fat, because it's kind of like having a lot of money in the bank.
Fiber	The nutritional value of the cardboard box that contains the good tasting food, like sugary cereal or cookies.
Food Chain	People worked hard to get to the top of the food chain. That means we can eat anything and everything. We shouldn't digress to eating plants.
Food Groups	There are four food groups: Fast, Frozen, Junk, and Instant.

Food Pyramid Like any pyramid scheme, you want to be at the top (i.e. eating desserts), not at the bottom (i.e. fruits and veggies).

Humanitarians Vegetarians eat vegetables. What do humanitarians eat?

Hunger A condition that prohibits you from dieting.

Indulges One who indulges bulges.

In Shape You're in shape. Round is a shape.

Junk Food First world term. People outside of the Western culture don't consider any food to be junk.

Life It's full of ups and pounds.

Obesity This is an ever expanding problem and too broad of a subject for a glossary.

Overweight Drought and famine resistant people.

Power Foods Food like beans. I can rip some powerful farts after eating beans.

Seconds Another serving of food. Never go back for seconds. Get it all the first time.

Success When you can look beyond food and look down and see your feet.

Successful Diet The triumph of mind over platter.

Thinner You can get thinner if you go to the paint store.

Vegetarian 1) A person that eats the food that food eats. 2) An old Indian word for bad hunter.

Waist A waist is a terrible thing to mind.

Weight Weight is relative and a function of gravity. For instance, you would weigh considerably less on the moon. Gravity is vastly different throughout the universe, so who can really say how much or little you really weigh? It all depends on where you are.

Weight
Watchers   People who watch other people diet.

Whole Foods   When eating, it is good to eat whole foods, like whole sheets of cake, whole bags of potato chips, and whole gallons of ice cream.

About the Author

Joe King, G.E.D, is a comedian posing as a gastroenteritis. He wrote The Contrarian Diet as dieting appeals to a very wide audience. He enjoys writing books and drinking, sometimes simultaneously. He lives alone.